"Those willing to delve into this unique work – even seasoned therapists – are lucky enough to embark on an initiatory journey by becoming part of the ongoing seminar this book brings to life. Its very form is moulded by the collaborative, highly respectful process of Solution-Focused Therapy and training, in which therapists and clients, trainers and trainees learn to learn from each other. In attending to how SFT techniques allow each of these parties to follow closely what the other says and how they say it, thereby achieving their respective goals, readers will surely find their view of therapy transformed."

Marika Moisseeff, psychiatrist and anthropologist; research fellow at the French National Center of Scientific Research

"Informed by the close, systematic observation of therapeutic encounters and a Wittgensteinian attention to context and language use, Solution-Focused Therapy is concerned less with the theoretical whys of hurtful repetition than with the concrete hows of hopeful change. The authors of this newly prefaced, analytically generous volume tack back-and-forth between grounded explanations of SFT's basic tools, comment-punctuated excerpts of actual therapy sessions in which they are put into effect, and insightful discussions of the larger issues they bring to the fore. In doing so, Steve de Shazer, Yvonne Dolan et al. provide an engaging yet comprehensive, multi-layered understanding of one of the most rigorous, demonstrably effective therapeutic approaches available today."

Michael Houseman, directeur d'études, École Pratique des Hautes Études (Paris)

"This text is a timely and valuable gathering together of the 'state of the art' of solution-focused brief therapy. Because of the simplicity of the chapters dealing with the core tenets of SFBT, it offers a valuable read for trainees who are working their way through the model. The first chapter is an excellent and simple summary of the whole model, with the verbatims demonstrating the principles. Likewise, experienced practitioners will find a pleasurable and thorough review of their knowledge of SFBT, with the level of detail just right."

Peter W. Cantwell, PhD lecturer, Swinburne University and Williams Road Family Therapy Centre, Victoria, Australia

"...essential reading...extremely valuable...must reading for SFBT therapists...a valuable resource for inquisitive practitioners....There is much to be learned about the specialized use of language in SFBT and this book provides an illuminating look into this topic..."

Wallace J. Gingerich, PhD, Families in Society: The Journal of Contemporary Social Services

More Than Miracles

Written by pioneering experts in the field, *More Than Miracles* remains the authoritative text on solution-focused brief therapy (SFBT). The final work of the world-renowned family therapists and original developers of SFBT, the late Steve de Shazer and Insoo Kim Berg, this comprehensive resource informs practitioners and students in how to apply this practical, internationally acclaimed approach.

With a new preface, this classic edition outlines the latest developments in the fields of family therapy, brief therapy, and psychotherapy training and practice. A succinct overview orients the reader to the current landscape of SFBT and provides three real-life case transcripts that illustrate the practical applications of SFBT techniques. The seminar format of the text allows readers to:

- sit in on surprising psychotherapy sessions
- eavesdrop on the authors' commentary about the sessions
- gain a comprehensive overview on the current state of SFBT
- review and understand the major tenets of SFBT
- learn specific interventions, including the miracle question and the reasons for asking it
- understand treatment applicability
- read actual session transcripts
- understand the "miracle scale"
- get insight into the unique relationship between Wittgenstein's philosophy and SFBT
- better understand SFBT and emotions
- examine misconceptions about SFBT
- *and more*

Suitable for both advanced practitioners and ambitious beginners, this book is the ideal resource for anyone seeking an in-depth understanding of the SFBT approach, the concepts that inform it, and the specific techniques that characterize its implementation.

Steve de Shazer, MSW, is co-developer of solution-focused brief therapy. He has published numerous journal articles and five groundbreaking books, which have been translated into 14 languages. He died in September 2005 in Vienna.

Yvonne Dolan is the author of five books and numerous articles and chapters on solution-focused brief therapy. She has been a psychotherapist for 30 years, lectures, and teaches seminars around the world on solution-focused brief therapy.

Routledge Mental Health Classic Edition

The *Routledge Mental Health Classic Edition* series celebrates Routledge's commitment to excellence within the field of mental health. These books are recognized as timeless classics covering a range of important issues, and continue to be recommended as key reading for professionals and students in the area. With a new introduction that explores what has changed since the books were first published, and why these books are as relevant now as ever, the series presents key ideas to a new generation.

Depression: The Evolution of Powerlessness (Classic Edition)
By Paul Gilbert

Human Nature and Suffering (Classic Edition)
By Paul Gilbert

Individuation and Narcissism (Classic Edition)
By Mario Jacoby

Shame and the Origins of Self-Esteem (Classic Edition)
By Mario Jacoby

Psychiatry and Religion (Classic Edition)
By Dinesh Bhugra

Therapeutic Trances: The Cooperation Principle in Ericksonian Hypnotherapy (Classic Edition)
By Stephen Gilligan

The Independent Mind in British Psychoanalysis (Classic Edition)
By Eric Rayner

More Than Miracles: The State of the Art of Solution-Focused Brief Therapy (Classic Edition)
By Steve de Shazer and Yvonne Dolan with Harry Korman, Terry Trepper, Eric McCollum, and Insoo Kim Berg

More Than Miracles

The State of the Art of Solution-Focused Brief Therapy

Classic Edition

Steve de Shazer, Yvonne Dolan
with Harry Korman, Terry Trepper,
Eric McCollum and
Insoo Kim Berg

Routledge
Taylor & Francis Group
NEW YORK AND LONDON

Classic edition published 2021
by Routledge
52 Vanderbilt Avenue, New York, NY 10017

and by Routledge
2 Park Square, Milton Park, Abingdon, Oxon OX14 4RN

Routledge is an imprint of the Taylor & Francis Group, an informa business

First edition published by Routledge 2007

Library of Congress Cataloging-in-Publication Data
Names: De Shazer, Steve, author.
Title: More than miracles: the state of the art of solution-focused brief therapy / Steve de Shazer [and five others].
Description: Classic edition. | New York, NY: Routledge, 2021. | Includes bibliographical references and index. |
Summary: "Written by pioneering experts in the field, More Than Miracles remains the authoritative text on Solution-focused Brief Therapy (SFBT). Suitable for both advanced practitioners and ambitious beginners, this book is the ideal resource for anyone seeking an in-depth understanding of the SFBT approach, the concepts that inform it, and the specific techniques that characterize its implementation" – Provided by publisher.
Identifiers: LCCN 2020040991 (print) | LCCN 2020040992 (ebook) | ISBN 9780367622435 (hardback) | ISBN 9780367646417 (paperback) | ISBN 9781003125600 (ebook)
Subjects: LCSH: Solution-focused brief therapy.
Classification: LCC RC489.S65 D38 2021 (print) | LCC RC489.S65 (ebook) | DDC 616.89/147–dc23
LC record available at https://lccn.loc.gov/2020040991
LC ebook record available at https://lccn.loc.gov/2020040992

ISBN: 978-0-367-62243-5 (hbk)
ISBN: 978-0-367-64641-7 (pbk)
ISBN: 978-1-003-12560-0 (ebk)

Typeset in Times New Roman
by Newgen Publishing UK

This book is dedicated to Steve de Shazer and Insoo Kim Berg with deep respect and appreciation.

Contents

About the Authors

Steve de Shazer, MSW, is co-developer of solution-focused brief therapy. He has published numerous journal articles and five groundbreaking books, which have been translated into 14 languages. He died in September 2005 in Vienna.

Yvonne Dolan is the author of five books and numerous articles and chapters on solution-focused brief therapy. She has been a psychotherapist for 30 years, lectures, and teaches seminars around the world on solution-focused brief therapy.

Harry Korman, MD, works in private practice in Malmö, Sweden, with families, children, adults, and couples. He supervises and teaches solution-focused therapy in a number of areas within the mental health field and parallel fields. He worked in child and adult psychiatry for 15 years before entering into private practice in 1996. He has published on solution-focused clinical work, on solution-focused theory, and on microanalysis of therapy dialogues. Most of his writings can be accessed for free at www.sikt.nu/publications/.

Terry S. Trepper, PhD, is Research Advisor for the Institute for Solution-Focused Therapy, and Professor Emeritus of Psychology, Purdue University Northwest. His scholarly and training interests include the evidence basis of solution-focused therapy, systemic and solution-focused approaches to treating substance abuse, and positive psychology.

Eric E. McCollum, PhD, is Professor Emeritus at Virginia Tech where he taught for 25 years prior to retiring in 2017. He is co-author of two additional books, *Family Solutions for Substance Abuse* with Terry Trepper, and *Couples Therapy for Domestic Violence* with Sandra Stith and Karen Rosen, and co-editor of *Solution-Focused Brief Therapy: A Handbook of Evidence-Based Practice* with Cynthia Franklin, Terry Trepper and Wallace J. Gingerich. His most recent book—*Mindfulness for Therapists: Practice for the Heart*—reflects his long-standing interest in mindfulness and its application in mental health and family therapy.

Insoo Kim Berg (1935–2007), was a world-renowned psychotherapist, lecturer, and author of ten groundbreaking psychotherapy books. Along with her husband, Steve de Shazer, she was the primary developer of the solution-focused brief therapy approach.

Preface to the Classic Edition

It has been 14 years since the publication of *More Than Miracles: The State of the Art of Solution-Focused Therapy* co-authored with our much esteemed friends and colleagues, Steve de Shazer, Insoo Kim Berg, Harry Korman, and Eric McCollum. Sadly, Steve passed away on September 11, 2005, a few months before the book's publication and Insoo less than a year and a half afterward, on January 10, 2007.

Whether seeking to optimize their implementation of the solution-focused brief therapy (SFBT) approach or gain a deeper understanding of the intellectually rigorous Wittgensteinian ideas that inform it, we predict that future generations of readers will find this new Routledge Classic Edition of *More Than Miracles: The State of the Art of the Solution-Focused Brief Therapy* to be as relevant, meaningful and satisfying today as when it was first written.

Characteristically modest and unassuming, original co-authors and SFBT developers de Shazer and Berg might have been surprised to see us begin this new Preface with a description of their unique personalities and how these contributed to the development of the approach and informs its continued evolution.

An iconoclastic creative genius, jazz saxophonist, abstract artist, social worker, and Wittgensteinian scholar, Steve de Shazer was precise and parsimonious with words, had a wry sense of humor and a soft-hearted, generous nature that belied his characteristically gruff communication style. He loved classical music, reading philosophy texts, the Milwaukee Brewers, a glass of good German or Belgian beer, cooking for his wife, Insoo, and taking long walks at the beginning, middle, and end of each day.

Insoo Kim Berg was intellectually brilliant, charismatic, caring, and dynamic. She was also multi-lingual. Raised in South Korea, Insoo spoke fluent Japanese as well as Korean and English. Originally coming to the United States to attend university, she went on to earn a graduate degree in social work, and stayed to co-develop the solution-focused approach. Living through the Korean war, Berg had witnessed horrific suffering, experienced severe hardship, and personal loss of loved ones. These experiences may account in part for her distinctive ability to be by turns soulfully reflective and empathic, yet highly practical in her approach to work and life.

Habitual early risers, Steve and Insoo seemed to be always working, tirelessly watching video tapes of recent SFBT sessions, seeing "live clients," sitting with the team behind the mirror during family therapy sessions at numerous social service and mental health agencies, writing scholarly articles and books, and meanwhile teaching seminars all over the world. While Berg and de Shazer had distinctly different personalities and unique interests, they shared several common traits that contributed significantly to the development of the SFBT and have continued to influence its evolution: a rigorous attention to detail, a desire to make things better for others and lessen human suffering, an appreciative recognition that real change can only occur in the present and future, a well-honed ability to stay fully present in the moment and make disciplined observations rather than subjective interpretations.

Over the course of our 25 year friendship, I (YD) observed a gradual evolution in the way de Shazer and Berg conceptualized essential aspects of the solution development process in SFBT. Based upon thousands of hours carefully observing SFBT sessions, Berg and de Shazer concluded that the words SFBT practitioners used to co-construct goals and develop solutions with their clients were important for the efficacy of the approach. Although SFBT sessions typically include a set of carefully worded questions, compliments, and scaling techniques, they strongly emphasized that the approach should never be conducted in a formulaic manner. Instead, every session must be guided by clients' individual needs, preferences, aspirations, and solutions highly individualized, derived from each client's unique experiential repertoire and life experiences. Throughout the SFBT process and particularly when formulating goals and developing solutions, SF therapists should be careful to incorporate clients' exact words.

As the years went by, Berg and de Shazer became increasingly attentive to subtle but important linguistic nuances that characterized the work of the best solution-focused practitioners and reached out to linguistic scholar Janet Bavelas for help in identifying and better understanding subtle but consistent patterns of communication specific to the SFBT approach evident in the work of advanced SFBT practitioners. This led to a series of microanalysis studies revealing unique features of SFBT that distinguished it from other behavioral approaches such as cognitive behavioral therapy (CBT) and motivational interviewing (MI) (see *Process Research*, below).

Research in Solution-Focused Brief Therapy

Since the publication of the first edition of *More Than Miracles: The State of the Art of Solution-Focused Brief Therapy*, there has been a great deal of both outcome and process empirical research that supports SFBT as an effective approach for most clinical populations and presenting problems. Further, SFBT is generally as or even more effective than other evidence-based approaches, but often obtains these results in fewer sessions, making it both clinically useful and cost-effective.

Origins as an Evidence-Based Approach

SFBT is one of the few approaches in psychotherapy that *began* as "evidence-based," as opposed to other models which are typically theory-driven. SFBT developers Steve de Shazer and Insoo Kim Berg and their team spent countless hours carefully observing real-life therapy sessions, meticulously noting any words or behavior on the part of the therapist that resulted in progress towards the client's stated goal. Language or behavior that reliably led to positive movement in the direction of the client's goal were preserved and incorporated into the solution-focused approach and those that did not were discarded (Lipchik, Derks, LaCourt, & Nunnally 2012).

Over the course of about ten years, a set of specific solution-focused interventions emerged primarily in the form of carefully worded questions, homework "experiments" and respectful compliments characterized by a general clinical style that could best be described as collegial, collaborative, and focused on solution development—as opposed to more interpretive, instructive, or confrontative, and focused on problem description. This *inductive* approach, rather than the more common *deductive* one that led to most other models, emerged to become what is now the standard practice of SFBT.

Randomized Clinical Trial and Meta-Analyses Outcome Research

There has been a great deal of empirical outcome research on SFBT, most of it occurring over the past 14 years (for a complete review of the scope of research in SFBT, see Kim, Jordan, Franklin, & Froerer, 2019; Kim, Smock, Trepper, McCollum, & Franklin, 2010). There have been over 150 randomized clinical trials (RCTs) with SFBT, and eight meta-analyses based on these. The conclusion of the eight meta-analyses, a number of systematic reviews of non-RCT studies, and the overall conclusion of the most recent scholarly works on SFBT, is that SFBT is an effective approach to the treatment of psychological problems, with effect sizes similar to other evidenced-based approaches, such as cognitive behavior therapy and interpersonal therapy, but that these effects are found in fewer average sessions, and using an approach style that is less intrusive than most other treatment models (Gingerich, Kim, & McDonald, 2012; Kim et al., 2019; Trepper & Franklin, 2012). That is, SFBT is an inherently collaborative approach and does not involve confrontation or interpretation. Given its equivalent effectiveness, shorter duration, and "user-friendly" collaborative approach, SFBT is considered to be an excellent first-choice evidenced-based psychotherapy approach for most psychological, behavioral, and relational problems.

The meta-analyses indicate that SFBT is effective with diverse clinical populations and different classes of presenting problems. For example, in terms of populations, SFBT was found to be effective in the treatment of children and adolescents (Carr, Hartnett, Brosnan, & Sharry, 2017; Gong & Hsu, 2017; Gong & Xu, 2015; Kim, 2008); and adults (Kim, 2008; Kim et al., 2015; Schmit, Schmit, & Lenz, 2016). In terms of presenting problems, SFBT has been shown to be effective in the treatment of child and adolescent behavioral problems (Carr et al., 2017; Gong & Hsu, 2017; Gong & Xu, 2015); externalizing behavioral problems, including conduct disorder and conflict management (Kim, 2008; Stams, Dekovic, Buist, & de Vries, 2006); internalizing behavioral problems, such as depression, anxiety, and self-esteem (Gong & Xu, 2015; Kim, 2008; Schmit, Schmit, & Lenz, 2016); and in providing behavioral and mental health support for medical and health-related problems (Zhang, Franklin, Currin-McCulloch, Park, & Kim, 2018). Also, a number of studies have shown SFBT to be effective for a variety of treatment-specific problems, including substance abuse (Kim, Brook, & Akin 2018; Smock et al, 2008); domestic violence (McCollum, Stith, & Thomsen 2011); burn victims (Wang, Li, Du, & Feng, 2016); and depression (Habibi, Ghaderi, Abedini, & Jamshidnejad, 2016). And a recent study (Kim, Brooke, & Akin, 2018) investigated the effectiveness of SFBT with parents of children with trauma-related problems and substance abuse for children in the child welfare system, where it was found that SFBT was as effective as the other evidence-based treatment approaches.

Process Research

There have been numerous studies examining the specific processes and mechanisms of change underlying the SFBT approach. In general, SFBT has been shown to have different mechanisms of change than other approaches, most notably CBT with which it is sometimes compared. Specifically in comparison to CBT and MI, SFBT has more positive content within the session with a concomitant tendency for clients to respond in kind (Jordan, Froerer, & Bavelas, 2013); SFBT therapists are more likely to use the specific language of the client to co-construct the goals and solutions (Korman, Bavelas, & De Jong 2013); and the SFBT interventions which focus on the strengths and resources of the clients tend to contribute to its successful outcomes (Beyebach, 2014; Franklin, Zhang, Froerer, & Johnson, 2017).

Much of the process research on SFBT has either used or been the result of studies utilizing the microanalysis of therapeutic communication and applied SFBT by Janet Bavelas and her colleagues (Bavelas, 2011; Bavelas & Jordan, 2014; Jordan & Bavelas, 2013; McKergow, 2013). This technique analyses the face-to-face dialogue and clinical interactions between therapist and client and examines the moment-by-moment details of therapeutic conversations. Microanalysis is one of the best empirical techniques to explore minute conversational data points which can be linked to immediate interactional and longer-term clinical outcomes.

A series of these microanalytic studies has begun to shed light on the actual process of SFBT and how it is different from other evidence-based approaches. Korman, Bavelas, and De Jong (2013) found that therapists *formulations* (comments directly following a statement by a client, sometimes in psychotherapy called paraphrasing or reflecting) were rarely neutral, and that SFBT therapists were more likely to preserve a higher proportion of clients' exact words with fewer therapist interpretations than CBT or MI therapists. Following up on the notion of lack of neutrality in clinical formulations, Jordan, Froerer, and Bavelas (2013) and Froerer and Jordan (2013) found that SFBT therapists were more likely to choose to discuss positive aspects of their clients' lives than CBT therapists. More significantly, they also found that positive talk by the therapist leads to positive talk by the client, and conversely negative talk by the therapist leads to more negative talk by the client.

An understanding of the language contribution to psychotherapy in general, and SFBT specifically, has led to some intriguing demonstrations of clinical applications. For example, Richmond, Jordan, Bishof, and Sauer (2014) demonstrated that clients taking solution-focused intake questionnaires described significantly more solutions, described fewer problems, and improved significantly before their first therapy session than those taking traditional problem-oriented intake procedures. Jordan (2014) describes the development and validation of a psychometrically sound assessment device, the Solution-Building Inventory (SBI), which, instead of measuring the problems and deficiencies assesses clients' ability to identify solutions, exceptions to problems, and hope. This instrument has utility both as a research tool and a clinical assessment device. Sánchez-Prada and Beyebach (2014) showed how therapists can use different language choices and dialogue deconstruction to help clients who report no improvement or worsening between sessions stop the negative spiral and begin showing improvement again.

As we write this new Preface, SFBT is being productively applied to an ever increasing variety of problems and social contexts including business, education, health care, social service and mental health. We predict that the efficacy, brevity, adaptability, and inherent respectfulness of this increasingly popular evidence-based approach will ensure its continued use and evolution for many years to come. We believe Steve and Insoo would be pleased to see the advancements made in SFBT over the past 14 years, and intrigued with the possibilities for its future.

Yvonne Dolan and Terry S. Trepper
Santa Fe, NM

References

Bavelas, J. (2011). From the lab to the therapy room: Microanalysis, co-construction, and solution-focused therapy. In C. Franklin, T. Trepper, W. J. Gingerich, & E. McCollum (Eds.), *Solution-Focused Brief Therapy: A handbook of evidence-based practice* (pp. 144–162). Oxford, UK: Oxford University Press.

Bavelas, J. B., & Jordan, S. S. (2014). Introduction to SFBT contributions to practice-oriented research. Part II: Changing the language of clinical practice. *Journal of Systemic Therapies*, 33(1), 30–32.

Beyebach, M. (2014). Change factors in solution-focused brief therapy: A review of the Salamanca studies. *Journal of Systemic Therapies*, 33(1), 62–77.

Carr, A., Hartnett, D., Brosnan, E., & Sharry, J. (2017). Parents plus systemic, solution-focused parent training programs: Description, review of the evidence base, and meta-analysis. *Family Process*, 56, 652–668.

Franklin, C., Zhang, A., Froerer, A., & Johnson, S. (2017). Solution-focused brief therapy: A systematic review and meta-summary of process research. *Journal of Marital and Family Therapy*, 43(1), 16–30.

Froerer, A. S., & Jordan, S. S. (2013). Identifying solution-building formulations through microanalysis. *Journal of Systemic Therapies*, 32(3), 60–73.
Gingerich, W.J., Kim, J. S., & MacDonald, A. J. (2012). Solution-focused brief therapy outcome research. In C. Franklin, T. S. Trepper, W. J. Gingerich, & E. E. McCollum (Eds.), *Solution-Focused Brief Therapy: A handbook of evidence-based practice* (pp. 95–111). New York: Oxford University Press.
Gong, H., & Hsu, W. (2017). The effectiveness of solution-focused group therapy in ethnic Chinese school settings: A meta-analysis. *International Journal of Group Psychotherapy*, 67, 383–409.
Gong, H., & Xu, W. (2015). A meta-analysis on the effectiveness of solution-focused brief therapy. *Studies of Psychology and Behavior*, 13, 799–803.
Habibi, M., Ghaderi, K., Abedini, S., & Jamshidnejad, N. (2016). The effectiveness of solution-focused brief therapy on reducing depression in women. *International Journal of Educational and Psychological Researches*, 2, 244–249.
Jordan, S. S. (2014). Asking different questions: Validation of the solution building inventory in a clinical sample. *Journal of Systemic Therapies*, 33(1), 78–88.
Jordan, S. S., & Bavelas, J. B. (2013). Introduction to SFBT contributions to practice-oriented research. Part I: Microanalysis of communication. *Journal of Systemic Therapies*, 32(3), 13–16.
Jordan, S. S., Froerer, A. S., & Bavelas, J. B. (2013). Microanalysis of positive and negative content in solution-focused brief therapy and cognitive behavioral therapy expert sessions. *Journal of Systemic Therapies*, 32(2), 46–59.
Korman, H., Bavelas, J. B., & De Jong, P. (2013). Microanalysis of formulations in solution-focused brief therapy, cognitive behavioral therapy, and motivational interviewing. *Journal of Systemic Therapies*, 32(3), 31–45.
Kim, J. S. (2008). Examining the effectiveness of solution-focused brief therapy: A meta-analysis. *Research on Social Work Practice*, 18(2), 107–116.
Kim, J. S., Brook, J., & Akin, B. A. (2018). Solution-Focused Brief Therapy with substance-using individuals: A randomized controlled trial study. *Research on Social Work Practice*, 28(4), 452–462.
Kim, J., Jordan, S. S., Franklin, C., & Froerer, A. (2019). Is solution-focused brief therapy evidence-based? An update 10 years later. *Families in Society: The Journal of Contemporary Social Services*, 100, 1–12.
Kim, J. S., Franklin, C., Zhang, Y., Liu, X., Qu, Y., & Chen, H. (2015). Solution-focused brief therapy in China: A meta-analysis. *Journal of Ethnic & Cultural Diversity in Social Work*, 24, 187–201.
Kim, J. S., Smock, S., Trepper, T., McCollum, E., & Franklin, C. (2010). Is solution-focused brief therapy evidence-based? *Families in Society: The Journal of Contemporary Social Services*, 91, 3894–4009.
Lipchik, E., Derks, J, LaCourt, M., & Nunnally, E. (2012). The evolution of Solution-Focused Brief Therapy. In C. Franklin, T. S. Trepper, W. J. Gingerich, & E. E. McCollum (Eds.), *Solution-Focused Brief Therapy: A handbook of evidence-based practice* (pp. 3–19). New York: Oxford University Press.

McCollum, E. E., Stith, S. M., & Thomsen, C. J. (2011). Solution-focused brief therapy in the conjoint couples treatment of intimate partner violence. In C. Franklin, T. S. Trepper, E. E. McCollum, & W. Gingerich (Eds.). *Solution-Focused Brief Therapy: A handbook of evidence-based practice* (pp. 183–195). New York: Oxford University Press.

McKergow, M. (2013). Fifty years of the Interactional View: An interview with Janet Bavelas. *InterAction*, 5(2), 92.

Richmond, C. J., Jordan, S. S., Bischof, G. H., & Sauer, E. M. (2014). Effects of solution-focused versus problem-focused intake questions on pre-treatment change. *Journal of Systemic Therapies*, 33(1), 33–47.

Schmit, E. L., Schmit, M. K., & Lenz, A. S. (2016). Meta-analysis of solution-focused brief therapy for treating symptoms of internalizing disorders. *Counseling Outcome Research and Evaluation*, 7(1), 21–39.

Smock, S. A., Trepper, T. S., Wetchler, J. L., McCollum, E. E., Ray, R., & Pierce, K. (2008). Solution-focused group therapy for level 1 substance abusers. *Journal of Marital and Family Therapy*, 34, 107–120.

Sánchez-Prada, A., & Beyebach, M. (2014). Solution-focused responses to "no improvement": A qualitative analysis of the deconstruction process. *Journal of Systemic Therapies*, 33(1), 48–61.

Stams, G. J. J., Dekovic, M., Buist, K., & de Vries, L. (2006). Effectiviteit van oplossings- gerichte korte therapie: Een meta-analyse [Efficacy of solution focused brief therapy: A meta-analysis]. *Gedragstherapie*, 39, 81–95. Retrieved from www.researchgate.net/publication/46670172_Effectiviteit_van_Oplossingsgerichte_Korte_Therapie_een_Meta-Analyse

Trepper, T. S., & Franklin, C. (2012). The future of research in Solution-Focused Brief Therapy. In C. Franklin, T. S. Trepper, W. J. Gingerich, & E. E. McCollum (Eds.), *Solution-Focused Brief Therapy: A handbook of evidence-based practice* (pp. 405–412). New York: Oxford University Press.

Wang, R., Li, X., Du, Y., & Feng, J. (2016) The effect of solution-focused nursing on the self-efficacy of burned patients. *International Journal of Nursing*, 35(15).

Zhang, A., Franklin, C., Currin-McCulloch, J., Park, S., & Kim, J. (2018). The effectiveness of strength-based, solution-focused brief therapy in medical settings: A systematic review and meta-analysis of randomized controlled trials. *Journal of Behavioral Medicine*, 41, 139–151.

Chapter 1

A Brief Overview

Solution-focused brief therapy (SFBT) is a future-focused, goal-directed approach to brief therapy developed initially by Insoo Kim Berg, Steve de Shazer, and their colleagues and clients at the Milwaukee Brief Family Therapy Center in the early 1980s. Developed inductively rather than deductively, SFBT is a highly disciplined, pragmatic approach rather than a theoretical one (Berg & Miller, 1992, Berg & Reuss, 1997; de Shazer, 1985, 1988, 1991, 1994). The developers observed hundreds of hours of therapy over the course of years, carefully noting the questions, behaviors, and emotions that led to clients conceptualizing and achieving viable, real-life solutions.

The questions that proved to be most consistently related to clients' reports of progress and solutions were carefully noted and painstakingly incorporated into the solution-focused approach, while those that did not were deliberately eliminated. Since then, the solution-focused brief therapy approach has become one of the leading schools of brief therapy throughout the world as well as a major influence in such divergent fields as business, social policy, and education.

MAJOR TENETS OF SFBT

SFBT is not theory based, but was pragmatically developed. One can clearly see the roots of SFBT in the early work of the Mental Research Institute in Palo Alto and of Milton H. Erickson; in Wittgensteinian philosophy; and in Buddhist thought. There are a number of tenets that serve as the guidelines for the practice of SFBT, and that both inform and characterize this approach.

If it isn't broken, don't fix it. This is the overarching tenet of SFBT. Theories, models, and philosophies of intervention are irrelevant if the client has already solved the problem. Nothing would seem more absurd than to intervene upon a situation that is already resolved. While this seems obvious, in reality there are some schools of psychotherapy that would encourage therapy in spite of improvement—for example, for "growth," to "solidify gains," or to get to "deeper meanings and structures." SFBT is antithetical to these. If there is no problem, there should be no therapy.

If it works, do more of it. Similar to the first tenet, this tenet continues the "hands-off" approach. If a client is in the process of solving a problem, the therapist's primary role should be to encourage the client to do more of what is already working. SFBT therapists do not judge the quality of a client's solutions, only whether a solution is effective. Following this, another related role for the therapist is helping the client maintain desired changes. This is accomplished by learning exactly how the client behaved or responded differently during periods of improvement. As a result of identifying what worked, the client is able to repeat this success and the solution further evolves.

If it's not working, do something different. To complete the obvious first three, this tenet suggests that no matter how good a solution might seem, if it does not work it is not a solution. An odd reality of human nature is the tendency to continue to try to solve problems by repeating the same things that have not worked in the past. This is especially true for psychotherapy, where many theories suggest that if the client does not improve (i.e., solve the problem), the fault rests with the client rather than the therapy or the theory. In SFBT, however, if a client does not complete a homework suggestion or experiment, the task is dropped, and something different is offered.

Small steps can lead to big changes. SFBT can be understood as a minimalist approach in which solution construction is typically accomplished in a series of small, manageable steps. It is assumed that once a small change has been made, it will lead to a series of further changes, which in turn lead to others, gradually resulting in a much larger systemic change without major disruption. Thus, small steps toward making things better help the client move gradually and gracefully forward to accomplish desired changes in their daily life and to subsequently be able to describe things as "better enough" for therapy to end.

The solution is not necessarily directly related to the problem. Whereas almost all other approaches to change have problem-leading-to-solution sequences, SFBT develops solutions by first eliciting a description of what will be different when the problem is resolved. The therapist and the client then work backward to accomplish this goal by carefully and thoroughly searching through the client's real-life experiences to identify times when portions of the desired solution description already exist or could potentially exist in the future. This leads to a model of therapy that spends very little or even no time on the origins or nature of the problem, the client's pathology, or analysis of dysfunctional interactions. While these factors may be interesting, and possibly could influence client behavior, SFBT focuses almost exclusively on the present and future. Viewed in this way, SFBT involves a true paradigm shift from other models of psychotherapy.

The language for solution development is different from that needed to describe a problem. The language of problems tends to be very different from that of solutions. As Ludwig Wittgenstein put it, "The world of the happy is quite another than that of the unhappy" (T, #6.43). Usually problem talk is negative and past-history focused (to describe the origins of the problem), and often suggests the permanence of a problem. The language of solutions, however, is usually more positive, hopeful, and future-focused, and suggests the transience of problems.

No problems happen all the time; there are always exceptions that can be utilized. This tenet, following the notion of problem transience, reflects the major intervention that is used continuously in SFBT, that is, that people always display exceptions to their problems, even small ones, and these exceptions can be utilized to make small changes.

The future is both created and negotiable. This tenet offers a powerful basis for the practice of SFBT. People are not seen as locked into a set of behaviors based on a history, a social stratum, or a psychological diagnosis. With strong social constructionist support, this tenet suggests that the future is a hopeful place, where people are the architects of their own destiny.

SFBT has its roots in the systems theory–based family therapies of the 1950s and 1960s and the work of Milton H. Erickson (Haley, 1973). Both Insoo Berg and Steve de Shazer had strong connections to the Mental Research Institute of Palo Alto, California. While the researchers at MRI focused primarily on problem formation and problem resolution (Watzlawick, Weakland, & Fish, 1974), the Brief Family Therapy Center in Milwaukee began exploring solutions. For a number of reasons, the current SFBT approach can be seen as a systemic therapy. First, SFBT therapists routinely treat systems because couples and families—as well as individuals—come in for treatment. SFBT therapists make their decision on who to see in a session based on who shows up; whoever walks in the door is seen. Second, SFBT is systemic because the solutions that are explored are interactional, that is, people's problems and their exceptions involve other people, very often family members, colleagues at work, or relationship partners and friends. Third, SFBT is systemic because once small changes begin to occur, larger changes often follow, and those larger changes are usually interactional and systemic.

THE ROLE OF THE THERAPIST

The role of the therapist in SFBT is different than in many other psychotherapeutic approaches. SFBT therapists accept that there is a hierarchy in the therapeutic arrangement, but this hierarchy tends to be more egalitarian and democratic than authoritarian. SFBT therapists almost never pass judgments about their clients, and avoid making any interpretations about the meanings behind their wants, needs, or behaviors. The therapist's role is viewed as trying to expand rather than limit options (Berg & Dolan, 2001). SFBT therapists lead the session, but they do so in a gentle way, "leading from one step behind" (Cantwell & Holmes, 1994, pp. 17-26). Instead of interpreting, cajoling, admonishing, or pushing, the therapist "taps on the shoulder" of the client (Berg & Dolan, 2001, p. 3), pointing out a different direction to consider.

THERAPEUTIC PRINCIPLES AND TECHNIQUES

Main Interventions

A positive, collegial, solution-focused stance. One of the most important aspects of SFBT is the general tenor and stance that is taken by the therapist. The overall attitude is positive, respectful, and hopeful. There is a general assumption that people have within them strong resiliencies, and can utilize these to make changes. Further, there is a core belief that most people have the strength, wisdom, and experience to effect change. What other models view as "resistance" is viewed in SFBT as (a) people's natural protective mechanisms, or realistic desire to be cautious and go slow, or (b) a therapist error, i.e., an intervention that does not fit the client's situation. All of these assumptions make for sessions that tend to feel collegial rather than hierarchical (although as noted earlier, SFBT therapists do "lead from behind"), and cooperative rather than adversarial.

Looking for previous solutions. SFBT therapists have learned that most people have previously solved many, many problems. This may have been at another time, another place, or in another situation. The problem may have also come back. The key is that the person had solved their problem, even if for a short time.

Looking for exceptions. Even when clients do not have a previous solution that can be repeated, most have recent examples of exceptions to their problem. An exception is thought of as a time when a problem could occur, but does not. The difference between a previous solution and an exception is small but significant. A previous solution is something that the family has tried on their own that has worked, but for some reason they have not continued this successful solution, and probably forgot about it. An exception is something that happens instead of the problem, usually without the client's intention or maybe even understanding.

Questions vs. directives or interpretations. Questions, of course, are an important communication element of all models of therapy. Therapists use questions often with all approaches, especially while taking a history, checking in at the beginning of a session, or finding out how a homework assignment went. SFBT therapists, however, make questions the *primary* communication tool, and as such they are an overarching intervention. SFBT therapists tend to make no interpretations, and rarely make direct challenges or confrontations to a client.

Present- and future-focused questions vs. past-oriented focus. The questions that are asked by SFBT therapists are almost always focused on the present or on the future. This reflects the basic belief that problems are best solved by focusing on what is already working, and how a client would like his or her life to be, rather than focusing on the past and the origin of problems.

Compliments. Compliments are another essential part of SFBT. Validating what clients are already doing well and acknowledging how difficult their problems are encourage the client to change while giving the message that the therapist has been listening (i.e., understands) and cares (Berg & Dolan, 2001). Compliments in therapy sessions can help to punctuate what the client is doing that is working.

Gentle nudging to do more of what is working. Once SFBT therapists have created a positive frame via compliments and then discovered some previous solutions and exceptions to the problem, they gently nudge the client to do more of what has previously worked, or to try changes brought up by the client—frequently called "an experiment." It is rare for an SFBT therapist to make a suggestion or assignment that is not based on the client's previous solutions or exceptions. It is always best if change ideas and assignments emanate from the client, at least indirectly during the conversation, rather than from the therapist, because the client is familiar with these behaviors.

Specific Interventions

Pre-session change. At the beginning or early in the first therapy session, SFBT therapists typically ask "What changes have you noticed that have happened or started to happen since you called to make the appointment for this session?" This question has three possible answers. First, the client may say that nothing has happened. In this case, the therapist simply goes on and begins the session by asking something like: "How can I be helpful to you today," or "What would need to happen today to make this a really useful session?"

The second possible answer is that things have started to change or get better. In this case, the therapist asks many questions about the changes that have started, requesting a lot of detail. This starts the process of "solution-talk," emphasizes the client's strengths and resiliencies from the beginning, and allows the therapist to ask: "So if these changes were to continue in this direction, would this be what you would like?" thus offering the beginning of a concrete, positive, and change-oriented goal.

The third possible answer is that things are about the same. The therapist could ask something like: "Is this unusual, that things have not gotten worse?" or "How have you all managed to keep things from getting worse?" These questions may lead to information about previous solutions and exceptions, and may move them into a solution-talk mode.

Solution-focused goals. As in many models of psychotherapy, clear, concrete, and specific goals are an important component of SFBT. Whenever possible, the therapist tries to elicit smaller goals rather than larger ones. More important, clients are encouraged to frame their goals as a solution, rather than the absence of a problem. For example, it is better to have as a goal "We want our son to talk nicer to us"—which would need to be described in greater detail—rather than "We would like our child to not curse at us." Also, if a goal is described in terms of its solution, it can be more easily scaled (see below).

Miracle question. Some clients have difficulty articulating any goal at all, much less a solution-focused goal. This is particularly true for multiproblem families, or clients for whom the problem is so severe, they feel that even the description of a goal somehow minimizes the magnitude of the problem and how overwhelming it feels. The miracle question is a way to ask for a client's goal that communicates respect for the immensity of the problem, yet at the same time leads to the client coming up with smaller, more manageable goals.

The precise language of the intervention may vary, but the basic wording is:

> I am going to ask you a rather strange question *[pause]*. The strange question is this: *[pause]* After we talk, you will go back to your work (home, school) and you will do whatever you need to do the rest of today, such as taking care of the children, cooking dinner, watching TV, giving the children a bath, and so on. It will become time to go to bed. Everybody in your household is quiet, and you are sleeping in peace. In the middle of the night, a miracle happens and the problem that prompted you to talk to me today is solved! But because this happens while you are sleeping, you have no way of knowing that there was an overnight miracle that solved the problem *[pause]*. So, when you wake up tomorrow morning, what might be the small change that will make you say to yourself, "Wow, something must have happened—the problem is gone!" (Berg & Dolan, 2001, p. 7)

Clients have a number of reactions to the question. They may seem puzzled. They may say they don't understand. They may smile. Usually, however, given enough time to ponder it, they come up with some very specific things that would be different when their problem is solved. The responses they give can then usually be taken as the goals of therapy. As such, their answers lead to a more detailed description of how they would like their life to be, which in turn can help elucidate their previous solutions and exceptions.

In therapy with couples, families, or work groups, the miracle question can be asked to individuals or to the group as a whole. If asked to individual members, each one would give his or her response to the question, and others might react to it. The

therapist would try to elicit support for each member's miracle. If the question is asked to the couple, family, or work group as a whole, members may "work on" their miracle together. The SFBT therapist, in trying to maintain a collaborative stance among family members, punctuates similar goals and supportive statements among family members. (See subsequent chapters for more details about the "miracle question" and its use.)

Scaling questions. Whether the client gives specific goals directly or via the miracle question, an important next intervention in SFBT is to scale each goal. The therapist asks the miracle question's scale: From 0-10 or from 1-10, where things were when the initial appointment was arranged, where things are now, and where they will be on the day after the miracle, i.e., when therapy is "successful." For example, with a couple for whom better communication is the goal:

THERAPIST: What I want to do now is scale the problem and the goal. Let's say a 1 is as bad as the problem ever could be, you never talk, only fight, or avoid each other all the time. And let's say a 10 is where you talk all the time, with perfect communication, never have a fight ever.

HUSBAND: That is pretty unrealistic.

THERAPIST: That would be the ideal. So where would you two say it was for you at its worst? Maybe right before you came in to see me.

WIFE: It was pretty bad . . . I don't know . . . I'd say a 2 or a 3.

HUSBAND: Yeah, I'd say a 2.

THERAPIST: Okay *[writing]* . . . a 2-3 for you, and a 2 for you. Now, tell me what you would be satisfied with when therapy is over and successful?

WIFE: I'd be happy with an 8.

HUSBAND: Well, of course I'd like a 10, but that is unrealistic. Yeah, I'd agree, an 8 would be good.

THERAPIST: What would you say it is right now?

WIFE: I would say it is a little better, because he is coming here with me, and I see that he is trying . . . I'd say maybe a 4?

HUSBAND: Well, that's nice to hear. I wouldn't have thought she'd put it that high. I would say it is a 5.

THERAPIST: Okay, a 4 for you, a 5 for you. And you both want it to be an 8 for therapy to be successful, right?

There are two major components of this intervention. First, it is a solution-focused assessment device, that is, if used at each session, the therapist and the clients have an ongoing measurement of their progress. Second, it is a powerful intervention in and of itself, because it allows the therapist to focus on previous solutions and exceptions, and to punctuate new changes as they occur. As with the changes made before the first session, there are three things that can happen between each session: (1) things can get better; (2) things can stay the same; (3) things can get worse.

If the scale goes up, and things get better from one session to the next, the therapist compliments the clients, then solicits extensive details describing how the clients were able to make such changes. This not only supports and solidifies the changes, but leads to the obvious nudge to "do more of the same." If things "stay the same," again, the clients can be complimented for maintaining their changes, or for not letting things get worse. "How did you keep it from going down?" the therapist might ask. It is interesting how often this question will lead to a description of changes the clients have made, in which case again the therapist can compliment and support and encourage more of that change.

THERAPIST: Mary, last week you were a 4 on the scale of good communications. I am wondering where you are this week?

WIFE: *[Pauses.]* I'd say a 5.

THERAPIST: A 5! Wow! Really, in just one week.

WIFE: Yes, I think we communicated better this week.

THERAPIST: How did you communicate better this week?

WIFE: Well, I think it was Rich. He seemed to try to listen to me more this week.

THERAPIST: That's great. Can you give me an example of when he listened to you more?

WIFE: Well, yes, yesterday for example. He usually calls me once a day at work, and . . .

THERAPIST: Sorry to interrupt, but did you say he calls you once a day? At work?

WIFE: Yes.

THERAPIST: I'm just a little surprised, because not all husbands call their wives every day.

WIFE: He has always done that.

THERAPIST: Is that something you like? That you wouldn't want him to change?

WIFE: Yes, for sure.

THERAPIST: Sorry, go on, you were telling me about yesterday when he called.

WIFE: Well, usually it is kind of a quick call. But I told him about some problems I was having, and he listened for a long time, seemed to care, gave me some good ideas. That was nice.

THERAPIST: So that was an example of how you would like it to be, where you can talk about something, a problem, and he listens and gives good ideas? Support?

WIFE: Yes.

THERAPIST: Rich, did you know that Mary liked your calling her and listening to her? That that made you two move up the scale, to her?

HUSBAND: Yeah, I guess so. I have really been trying this week.

THERAPIST: That's great. What else have you done to try to make the communication better this week?

This example shows how going over the scale with the couple served as a vehicle for finding the clients' progress. The therapist gathered more and more information about the small changes the clients had made on their own, that led to an improvement on the scale. This would naturally lead to the therapist suggesting that the couple continue to do the things that are working, in this case for the husband to continue calling her, and continue to engage in the active listening that she found so helpful. (See subsequent chapters for more details about "scaling questions.")

Constructing solutions and exceptions. The SFBT therapist spends most of the session listening attentively for signs of previous solutions, exceptions, and goals. When these come out, the therapist punctuates them with enthusiasm and support. The therapist then works to keep the solution-talk in the forefront. This, of course, requires a whole range of different skills than those used in traditional problem-focused therapies. Whereas the problem-focused therapist is concerned with missing signs of what has caused or is maintaining a problem, the SFBT therapist is concerned with missing signs of progress and solution.

MOTHER: She always just ignores me, acts like I'm not there, comes home from school, just runs into her room; who knows what she is doing in there.

DAUGHTER: You say we fight all the time, so I just go in my room so we don't fight.

MOTHER: See? She admits she just tries to avoid me. I don't know why she can't just come home and talk to me a little about school or something, like she used to.

THERAPIST: Wait a second, when did she "use to"? Anita, when did you used to come home and tell your mom about school?

DAUGHTER: I did that a lot; last semester I did.

THERAPIST: Can you give me an example of the last time you did that?

MOTHER: I can tell you, it was last week, actually. She was all excited about her science project getting chosen.

THERAPIST: Tell me more, what day was that . . . ?

MOTHER: I think last Wednesday.

THERAPIST: And she came home . . .

MOTHER: She came home all excited.

THERAPIST: What were you doing?

MOTHER: I think the usual, I was getting dinner ready. And she came in all excited, and I asked her what was up, and she told me her science project was chosen for the display at school.

THERAPIST: Wow, that is quite an honor.

MOTHER: It is.

THERAPIST: So then what happened?

MOTHER: Well, we talked about it; she told me all about it.

THERAPIST: Anita, do you remember this?

DAUGHTER: Sure, it was only last week. I was pretty happy.

THERAPIST: And would you say that this was a nice talk, a nice talk between you two?

DAUGHTER: Sure. That's what I mean; I don't always go in my room.

THERAPIST: Was there anything different about that time, last week, that made it easier to talk to each other?

MOTHER: Well, she was excited.

DAUGHTER: My mom listened, wasn't doing anything else.

THERAPIST: Wow, this is a great example, thank you. Let me ask this, if it were like that more often, where Anita talked to you about things that were interesting and important to her, and where Mom, you listened to her completely without doing other things, is that what you two mean by better communication?

DAUGHTER: Yeah, exactly.

MOTHER: Yes.

In this example, the therapist did a number of things. First, she listened carefully for an exception to the problem, a time when the problem could have happened but it did not. Second, she punctuated that exception by repeating it, emphasizing it, getting more details about it, and congratulating them on it. Third, she connected the exception to their goal (or miracle) by asking the question: If this exception were to occur more often, would your goal be reached?

Coping questions. If a client reports that the problem is not better, the therapist may sometimes ask coping questions, such as, for example, "How have you managed to prevent it from getting worse?" or "This sounds hard—how are you managing to cope with this to the degree that you are?"

Is there anything I forgot to ask? Before taking a break and reconvening or alternatively, sometime during the session, the therapist asks the client, "Is there anything I forgot to ask?" or "Is there something else I need to know?"

Taking a break and reconvening. Many models of family therapy have encouraged therapists to take a break toward the end of the session. Usually this involves a conversation between the therapist and a team of colleagues or a supervision team who have been watching the session and who give feedback and suggestions to the therapist. In SFBT, therapists are also encouraged to take a break near the session end. If there is a team, they give the therapist feedback, a list of compliments for the family, and some suggestions for interventions based on the clients' strengths, previous solutions, or exceptions. If there is a not a team available, the therapist will still take a break to collect his or her thoughts, and then come up with compliments and ideas for possible experiments. When the therapist returns to the session, he or she can offer the family compliments.

THERAPIST: I just wanted to tell you, the team was really impressed with you two this week. They wanted me to tell you that, Mom, thcy thought you really seem to care a lot about your daughter. It is really hard to be a mom, and you seem so focused, and clear how much you love her and how you want to help her. They were impressed that you came to the session today, in spite of work and having a sick child at home. Anita, the team also wanted to compliment you on your commitment to making the family better. They wanted me to tell you how bright and articulate they think you are, and what a good "scientist" you are! Yes, that you seem to be really aware of what small, little things that happen in your family might make a difference . . . That is what scientists do, they observe things that seem to change things, no matter how small. Anyway, they were impressed with you two a lot!

DAUGHTER: *[Seeming pleased.]* Wow, thanks!

Experiments and homework assignments. While many models of psychotherapy use intersession homework assignments to solidify changes begun during therapy, most of the time the homework is assigned by the therapist. In SFBT, therapists frequently end the session by suggesting a possible experiment for the client to try between sessions if they so choose. These experiments are based on something the client is already doing (exceptions), thinking, feeling, etc. that is heading them in the direction of their goal. Alternately, homework is sometimes designed by the client. Both approaches follow the basic philosophy that what emanates from the client is better than if it were to come from the therapist. This is true for a number of reasons. First, what is suggested by the client, directly or indirectly, is familiar. One of the main reasons homework is not completed in other models is that it is foreign to the family, thus it takes more thinking and work to accomplish (usually thought of as "resistance"). Second, clients usually assign themselves either more of what has worked already for them (a previous solution) or something they really want to do. In both cases, the homework is more tied to their own goals and solutions. Third, creating their own homework assignments reduces clients' natural tendency to "resist" outside intervention, no matter how good the intention. While SFBT does not focus on resistance (and, in fact, views this phenomenon as a natural, protective process that people use to move slowly and cautiously into change rather than as evidence of psychopathology), certainly when clients initiate their own homework, there is a greater likelihood of success.

THERAPIST: Before we end today, I would like for you two to think about a homework assignment. If you were to give yourselves a homework assignment this week, what would it be?

DAUGHTER: Maybe that we talk more?

THERAPIST: Can you tell me more?

DAUGHTER: Well, that I try to talk to her more when I come home from school. And that she stops what she is doing and listens.

THERAPIST: I like that. You know why? Because it is what you two were starting to do last week. Mom, what do you think? Is that a good homework assignment?

MOTHER: Yeah, that's good.

THERAPIST: So let's make this clear. Anita will try to talk to you more when she comes home from school. And you will put down what you are doing, if you can, and listen and talk to her about what she is talking to you about. Anything else? Anything you want to add?

MOTHER: No, that's good. I just need to stop what I was doing; I think it is important to listen to her.

THERAPIST: Well, that sure seemed to work for you two last week. Okay, so that's the assignment. We'll see how it went next time.

A couple of points should be emphasized here: First, the mother and daughter were asked to make their own assignment rather than have one imposed on them by the therapist. Second, what they assigned themselves flowed naturally from their previous solution and exceptions from the week before. This is very common and is encouraged by SFBT therapists. However, even if the clients suggested an assignment that was not based on solutions and exceptions to the problem, the therapist would most likely support it. What is preeminent is that the assignments come from the clients.

So, what is better, even a little bit, since the last time we met? At the start of each session after the first one the therapist will usually ask about progress, about what has been better during the interval. Many clients will report that there have been some noticeable improvements. The therapist will help the client describe these changes in as much detail as possible. Of course some clients will report that things have remained the same or have become worse. This will lead the therapist to explore how the client has managed to keep things from becoming worse, or, if worse, what the client did to prevent things from becoming *much* worse. Whatever the client has done to prevent things for worsening is then the focus and a source for compliments and perhaps for an experiment, because whatever they did they should continue doing. During the session, usually after there has been a lot of talk about what is better, the therapist will ask the client to rate himself or herself on the progress (toward solution) scale. Of course when the rating is higher than the previous session's, the therapist will compliment this progress and help the client figure out how to maintain the improvement.

At some point during the session—possibly at the beginning, perhaps later in the session—the therapist will check, frequently indirectly, on how the assignment went. If the client did the assignment, and it "worked"—that is, it helped the client move toward his or her goals—the therapist will offer a compliment. If the client did not do the assignment, the therapist usually drops it, or asks what was done instead that was better.

One difference between SFBT and other homework-driven models, such as cognitive-behavioral therapy, is that the homework itself is not required for change per se, so not completing an assignment is not addressed. If the client does not complete an assignment it is assumed that: (a) something realistic got in the way of its completion, such as work or illness; (b) the client did not find the assignment useful; (c) the assignment was not relevant during the interval between sessions. In any case, there is no fault assigned. If the client did the assignment but things did not improve or became worse, the therapist handles this in the same way he or she would when problems stay the same or become worse in general.

TREATMENT APPLICABILITY

Solution-focused therapy is one of the most popular and widely used models of therapy in the world. Because it is based on the concept of resiliency, and on clients' own previous solutions and exceptions to their own problems, it is applicable to all problems, and indeed has been applied to a wide range of problems seen by clinicians. These include family therapy (McCollum & Trepper, 2001); couples therapy (Weiner-Davis, 1993); treatment of sexual abuse (Dolan, 1991); treatment of substance abuse (Berg & Miller, 1992; de Shazer & Isebaert, 2003); and treatment of schizophrenia (Eakes, Walsh, Markowski, Cain, & Swanson, 1997). There have been self-help books written from a solution-focused perspective (Dolan, 1998), and the solution-focused approach has been applied beyond traditional psychotherapy practice to include interventions in social service agencies (Pichot & Dolan, 2003), educational settings and model schools (Rhodes & Ajmal, 2001), and business systems (Caufman, 2001).

RESEARCH ON THE EFFECTIVENESS OF SOLUTION-FOCUSED BRIEF THERAPY

Considering the wide use of SFBT, both in clinical practice and in other social systems, it is unfortunate that more empirical research has not been done on its effectiveness. In the most thorough review to date, Gingerich and Eisengart (2000) review 15 empirical studies on SFBT effectiveness. Of the five studies that were considered well-controlled, four were found to be superior to no treatment or treatment as usual; the fifth was found to be equal to a known intervention, interpersonal psychotherapy for depression. The findings for the remaining ten studies, which were not considered as well-controlled or which had methodological problems, all support SFBT's effectiveness. Gingerich and Eisengart conclude that, while this review provides preliminary support for SFBT's effectiveness, more and better-controlled studies are necessary.

SUMMARY

SFBT is a paradigm shift from the traditional psychotherapy focus on problem formation and problem resolution that underlies almost all psychotherapy approaches since Freud. Instead, SFBT draws upon clients' strengths and resiliencies by focusing on their own previous or conceptualized solutions and exceptions to their problems, and then, through a series of interventions, encouraging the clients to do more of those behaviors. SFBT can be applied to a myriad of family-related problems. SFBT, while deceptively easy to learn, like all therapies, requires great skill to reach a level of proficiency. While the preliminary research on the effectiveness of SFBT has been positive, clearly more research, especially clinical trial studies, are needed.

Chapter 2

I Feel Really Confused

The client, Margaret, is an attractive young woman in her early 20s. The person she refers to as "Harry" is Harry Korman, MD, Margaret's primary therapist. Yvonne Dolan is the consulting therapist in this session.

YVONNE: I really appreciate you seeing me. You don't even know me.

MARGARET: *[Laughs.]*

YVONNE: What would need to happen here so that when you leave you could say it was worth your time, the time you spent . . . that it was worthwhile for you?

MARGARET: I appreciate Harry a lot because he makes me think myself, you know. Do you understand what I mean?

YVONNE: I think so.

MARGARET: Yeah. And, I think I get a little bit farther along every time I see him because it's just "Oh, okay, maybe I have to think about that and that."

YVONNE: So seeing Harry makes a difference?

MARGARET: Yeah, I think so.

YVONNE: Would it be helpful if we spent this session talking about how seeing Harry makes a difference?

MARGARET: Well, ah, maybe . . . I don't know if that's necessary.

YVONNE: Mmm-hmm. Mmm-hmm. So let me see if I understand. Um, when I asked you, you know, what would be useful, you said that it's helpful for you when you think for yourself. That's a good thing.

MARGARET: Yeah. Yeah.

YVONNE: So, at the end of our time, you're walking out the door. How would we have spent the time so that you'd be able to say, "Well, I got something from it"?

MARGARET: *[Laughs.]* Yeah. Right now I think I need help how I should handle a situation I'm in right now.

YVONNE: Mmm-hmm.

MARGARET: And, I feel really confused. I don't know what to do.

As Wittgenstein puts it: "A . . . problem has the form: 'I don't know my way about'" (PI, #123). The conversation "simply puts everything before us, and neither explains nor deduces anything—since everything lies open to view there is nothing to explain" (PI, #126).

YVONNE: Mmm-hmm. So you might have an idea about how to handle it?

Right from the beginning of this session, the therapist responds primarily with questions. Is a reliance on questions fundamental to the SFBT approach or a matter of personal style? Would it be possible to do SFBT well without relying on questions?

What is really important here is what the client says in response to the therapist's questions. Watching Insoo Kim Berg, Steve de Shazer, Luc Isebaert, Yvonne Dolan, and others, questions seem to be very much part of the approach. Of course, if these kinds of client responses can be developed without questions, that would be great.

MARGARET: Uh, hmm. I don't know really. I don't know if Harry told you . . .

In order to be useful, a technique needs to go through the filter of that therapist's immediate experience in that room, and of course their personality and background, so that it becomes a highly personalized, meaningful response to the person at that exact moment in the session, not just the session in general, but that exact moment. How do you do this?

You have to use the client's exact words as much as possible, and focus on only what he has already told you.

YVONNE: No, no.

MARGARET: . . . anything about me or . . .

YVONNE: Well, what I preferred . . .

MARGARET: Yeah.

YVONNE: . . . was to just ask you.

MARGARET: Okay.

YVONNE: So he would have been willing to, I suppose . . .

MARGARET: *[Laughs.]*

YVONNE: . . . if he had your permission. but I thought I would ask you . . .

MARGARET: Okay. Okay.

YVONNE: . . . what needed to happen? And so, if you and I did a good job today . . . when you leave, you would have perhaps an idea about this situation that was useful?

MARGARET: Yeah. Yeah.

YVONNE: Well . . . please tell me what I need to know in order to be helpful to the degree you're comfortable because I know you don't know me.

MARGARET: *[Laughs.]*

YVONNE: To the degree you're comfortable doing that.

MARGARET: Yeah. Okay. Um. I'm not so good at English, but maybe—

YVONNE: Oh, Margaret, I think you're very good at English. My Swedish and my Danish are nonexistent! So the fact that you speak any English, I'm very impressed.

MARGARET: Okay.

YVONNE: How did you learn English, by the way?

MARGARET: Uh, first in school but then I've been traveling a little bit, so . . .

YVONNE: Where?

MARGARET: I've been in Australia.

About history-taking, oftentimes beginning students don't realize that what clients don't talk about is just as important a source of information as what they do talk about. How does someone teach a student to listen to what is missing? A not-knowing stance helps people learn this. Furthermore, it helps to know about child development, life experience. For example, how a mother talks about a baby tells a lot about the bond between them.

YVONNE: Oh, my goodness.

MARGARET: Asia, U.S.A., New Zealand.

YVONNE: Wow. No wonder. Do you like to travel?

MARGARET: I do understand [English]. Yeah, I do.

YVONNE: Wow.

MARGARET: Okay, so I will try. I had this relationship with a guy for three years and we were both drug addicts.

YVONNE: Hmm.

MARGARET: Yeah. And it was a lot of fights and it was really not easy to live with him. So in April, I went to this family who works with drug addicts and . . .

YVONNE: Oh.

MARGARET: . . . people with problems.

YVONNE: Mmm-hmm. How did you decide to do that?

MARGARET: Oh, first of all, I . . . all my days was just . . . I was so afraid for everything and I used a lot of drugs.

YVONNE: So you decided to take some action, to go to this family?

MARGARET: Yeah.

YVONNE: Wow. And that was in April?

MARGARET: Yeah.

YVONNE: Hmm. So you took a step?

MARGARET: Yeah. Yeah.

YVONNE: Hmm.

MARGARET: And I also left this man.

YVONNE: Also in April?

MARGARET: Yeah. Yeah. But now my problem is I can't forget him and *[sighs]* and I have had contact with him on the phone again.

YVONNE: Mmm-hmm.

MARGARET: And the family I live with doesn't know that.

She is living with this family and she is lying to them, and is in danger of going back to this guy with whom she used drugs and who abused her, and yet you do not confront this directly?

In fact, I was horrified at the danger of her going back, but because I have worked with addicts I know that taking a moral high ground and confronting her, e.g., "How do you think this would make your family feel if they knew you were lying to them," is not going to be helpful in motivating her to resist the temptation to use drugs and fall back into an abusive relationship. Instead, I go on to ask her a series of questions, and in her answers she subsequently proceeds to deliver her own self-motivating lecture about the reasons it would not be good for her to return to the abusive boyfriend or to using drugs. Asking clients in situations such as this what someone else who cares about her would say allows her by answering to put the concerns into her own words and thereby make them much more appropriate and effective than a lecture to her.

YVONNE: Hmm.

MARGARET: And it's a really big problem for me because I'm afraid that I will go back to him and then I . . . then I don't know if it will work out.

YVONNE: So, um, help me understand this. So you're afraid you will go back to him and you don't know if it will work out with him or with the family or for you or . . . ?

MARGARET: Um. *[Laughs.]* I guess for me. But also, I will hurt my family a lot. I know that everybody is so afraid that I will go back to him.

YVONNE: So this family really cares about you?

MARGARET: Yeah. Yeah.

YVONNE: Oh. And, I guess if they're afraid, it would mean they don't want anything bad to happen to you?

Instead of implying that she is a bad person for being tempted to go back, the therapist emphasizes the fact that she has managed in the past to make good decisions and so presumably has the potential to do so again.

MARGARET: Yeah, that's right.

YVONNE: Wow. How long have you known this family? Just since April or before?

MARGARET: No, um, I knew the Rowson's since I was born because she's a friend of my dad's. We didn't have—we hadn't this contact for all these years.

YVONNE: Mmm-hmm.

MARGARET: Yeah.

YVONNE: So, these are people who care about you.

MARGARET: Yeah, and I have my father and my mom. And I think they will be really, really sad if I go back.

YVONNE: What do you think they would be sad about?

MARGARET: Well, um, first of all, I think they just really don't think he's good for me.

YVONNE: Mmm-hmm.

MARGARET: And he beat me.

YVONNE: Oh my God.

MARGARET: Yep. And my father also lives in [name of town] so he really tried to have a conversation with Paul.

YVONNE: I see.

MARGARET: Yeah. And he tried to help us, but didn't work out.

YVONNE: Mmm-hmm.

MARGARET: And I think in a way he's like a drug for me. I can't . . . I can't stop thinking of him.

Wittgenstein reminds us that a feeling described as "like a drug for me" and "thinking" are each an "inner process [that] stand in need of outward criteria" (PI, #580) and now the question around feelings and thoughts is "How is this manifested in behavior" (PI, #579)? " 'But the inner is hidden from me'—isn't that just as vague as the concept of 'inner'? (For just consider: the inner after all is sensations + thought + images + mood + intention, and so on)" (LWPP, #959).

YVONNE: Mmm-hmm.

MARGARET: Even though I know that this is not good.

YVONNE: Mmm-hmm. So, you . . . you say you know it's not good. You decided it's not good to be with him and yet you want to be with him?

MARGARET: Yep. I think I still hope that it will work out, that he will change and . . .

YVONNE: So let me see if I understand this: In April, I mean you did two really big things it seems like. You moved . . .

MARGARET: Mmm-hmm.

YVONNE: . . . in with this family. You left the man who was beating you.

MARGARET: Yeah.

YVONNE: What about drugs? Did you change that, too?

MARGARET: Yeah.

YVONNE: How did you do it?

MARGARET: Well, I guess I just decided that this is . . . it has to have a stop. It was like I chose not using drugs at all or just . . . I knew that I would die . . .

YVONNE: Wow.

MARGARET: . . . if I go on like this. So . . .

YVONNE: So you really . . . you thought you could die?

MARGARET: Yeah.

YVONNE: Did that make a difference?

MARGARET: Yeah.

YVONNE: Uh-huh.

MARGARET: Before I'd been really, really ill and . . . and very thin.

YVONNE: Mmm-hmm.

MARGARET: Yeah. But I didn't care much then . . . just like "It doesn't matter."

YVONNE: Mmm-hmm. Mmm-hmm. How'd you get from there to, you know, realizing you didn't want to die?

MARGARET: Oh, well, I had my parents and I had a lot of friends (about) who I always felt like: "It doesn't matter for them because I'm just a big problem." But, I realized that they really cared. They really loved me.

YVONNE: And you really realized that?

MARGARET: Yeah.

YVONNE: How did that feeling come through for you so you knew that?

MARGARET: Um. Because they never gave up.

YVONNE: Wow.

MARGARET: Yeah. They were always there.

YVONNE: So you could just . . . because they were there, you knew somehow?

MARGARET: Yeah, they cared a lot.

YVONNE: I'm very interested because you say he's kind of like a drug.

MARGARET: Mmm-hmm.

YVONNE: How's he like a drug for you?

Why did you ask her this? It would seem you are asking her about the problem?

She has told me she wants to understand her situation so as to make a decision, and I am trying to be faithful to this goal she has set by helping her clarify what she thinks about the situation. A propo of Wittgenstein, I want to be faithful to understanding what she knows—I want to understand and I want her to understand what she already knows about this situation by exploring the details. For example, when someone says "He is like a drug for me," it could mean many different things for different clients. A word carries a halo of meaning, as Wittgenstein says, and there is a danger of making false assumptions based upon what we think the other person means. There is a danger in assuming we know what the client means when very likely we do not. For example, "like a drug" might suggest a "high." But in her case, he is like a drug that renders her incompetent. Such a simple sentence.

Furthermore, asking her how he is a drug for her allows her to make a case for why she should not go back to him.

MARGARET: Um. Well, when we were together I was—I didn't think that I could do anything by myself.

YVONNE: That makes sense.

MARGARET: Yeah.

YVONNE: How did you find a way to break away? That's pretty incredible. You gave up two things at the same time, it sounds like. Both in April?

MARGARET: Yeah.

YVONNE: Drugs and your relationship.

MARGARET: I actually went to this family last year also.

YVONNE: Mmm-hmm.

MARGARET: And I decided then to stop with the drugs because I was in the hospital. My heart stopped.

YVONNE: Oh my God.

MARGARET: That was for the fifth time.

YVONNE: Oh!

MARGARET: And I decided . . .

YVONNE: Yes?

MARGARET: ". . . okay, I have to stop." But, I still had Paul with me. So, I decided to go back to him and then after just a couple of weeks I started with the drugs again.

YVONNE: Hmm.

MARGARET: So . . .

YVONNE: Is that why you worried about going back to him?

MARGARET: I don't know really. Because I had this hope that I know that he's not on drugs now.

YVONNE: Mmm hmm.

MARGARET: And, I think maybe that we could, could have a relationship without drugs.

YVONNE: Mmm-hmm.

MARGARET: But I'm afraid that I won't use my own head anymore and . . .

YVONNE: Mmm-hmm. Mmm-hmm.

MARGARET: I'm afraid that I can't . . . if it was start all over again . . .

YVONNE: Hmm. Yeah.

MARGARET: What shall I do?

YVONNE: Yeah.

MARGARET: Am I strong enough to walk away? I don't think I am. So, that's why I'm worried.

YVONNE: Mmm-hmm . . . *[Pauses.]* How soon do you need to make a decision?

MARGARET: I think pretty soon because I don't want to leave everything here and just go away. And, I'm afraid if I don't do anything, that's what I will do. And then I end up in [name of city] where I lived before.

YVONNE: Mmm-hmm.

MARGARET: And I was selling drugs also. So, now I would be with the people who are not good for me at all.

YVONNE: Mmm-hmm. Mmm-hmm.

MARGARET: Yeah.

YVONNE: So, this is kind of a funny question.

MARGARET: Mmm-hmm.

YVONNE: If you had a scale and zero was you didn't even think about any decision . . .

MARGARET: Mmm-hmm.

YVONNE: . . . and 10 was you were completely confident that you'll make the right decision, where are you right now?

Why did you ask her about confidence here rather than asking her directly about making the decision?

Because she has already said in reference to her boyfriend being like a drug, that in that situation she didn't feel like she could do anything, she didn't listen to herself or believe in herself, and by implication she had no confidence in herself. Believing in herself is very crucial to the solution because in describing the trouble she is in she characterizes it as not believing in herself and not having confidence that if she gets into the situation she will be able to get out of it again.

MARGARET: I think I'm on my way to making the wrong decisions, so maybe 4 or something.

YVONNE: So what number of confidence would you need in order to trust that you could make the right decision for you?

MARGARET: I think maybe 7 or 8.

YVONNE: Maybe a 7 or an 8. And you're at 4 now. Has Harry ever asked you the miracle question?

MARGARET: Yeah. *[Laughs.]*

YVONNE: Well, do you mind if I ask you it again?

Some therapists might at this point say to her, "Let's make a decision"; why don't you do that?

If making a productive decision were simple, she would have already done it. Since she has not, I focus first on what it would take for her to be confident that she can now make a good decision. She has let us know that she has to make a decision soon, but fears making a wrong decision.

MARGARET: No.

In answering these scaling questions, she's gradually building a case for herself against deciding to go back to the boyfriend and the drugs.

My clients are nowhere near knowing drugs are bad for them. What do you do with people who are not as smart as this client is? Questions about how the client sees other people seeing them can be useful. In many situations such as this somebody is nagging the client about drug use so a question might be asked regarding how would this person be convinced to stop nagging? Of course, when the client is somehow involuntary and does not want to stop using drugs, then "not knowing that drugs are bad" is a reasonable deference strategy. Only if they want to achieve something else and stopping drugs makes achieving that goal more likely will they find stopping drugs is a reasonable, logical thing to do.

YVONNE: Sometimes it helps me understand.

MARGARET: Okay.

YVONNE: Do you have your own room with this family?

MARGARET: Yeah. *[Laughs.]*

YVONNE: Do you like that?

MARGARET: Yeah.

YVONNE: Sometimes it can be really important to have one's own room.

MARGARET: Yeah. Yeah.

YVONNE: Let's suppose that tonight you go back there and you do whatever you normally do to get ready for bed.

MARGARET: Yeah.

YVONNE: And you're . . . you're good to yourself. You know. You do whatever it is that makes you comfortable and you get into bed. Are you a good sleeper?

MARGARET: No, not right now, but— *[Laughs.]*

YVONNE: Okay. So let's imagine that maybe at first you have a little trouble sleeping.

MARGARET: Yeah.

YVONNE: Because that's kind of normal right now. But somehow or other, you eventually drift off to sleep.

MARGARET: Mmm-hmm.

YVONNE: And I don't know if you notice that you're falling off to sleep or maybe you just fall asleep. But, somehow it's a good sleep.

MARGARET: Mmm-hmm.

YVONNE: And sometime when you're sleeping, you're warm enough, you're not too cool. You're not too warm. You're just kind of right. Maybe you're having a dream, maybe not. But somehow deep inside you, something shifts. And I don't know whether it's something with your confidence or maybe it's some wisdom you've been kind of storing up all along, or maybe it's almost like an angel gives you a little blessing. I don't know what it is, but something shifts. And you know how to make the right decision. You know how to make the decision that's best for you. But you don't know that happened because you're asleep.

And so eventually, you wake up. You're going through your day. But your confidence now is more like a 7 or an 8. Maybe 7½ even. What would your family notice? What would you notice that would make you say, "Hmm, it's not a 4 anymore. It's a 7 or 8"? What do you think you'd notice that would let you know it was at a 7 or maybe even an 8? What will be different?

MARGARET: Um, first of all, I think he's not the first thing on my mind.

You ask the miracle question in a sort of odd way, talking about being "not too hot" and "not too cold," and either "drifting off to sleep without realizing it" or having some trouble first and then falling asleep. Is this due to an integration of your Ericksonian background with SFBT?

Clients are better able to respond to the miracle question from a context of imagined comfort and security, and I wanted her comfortable, so I specified that she would feel neither too hot nor too cold. Of course there are other ways to imply a context of comfort and security without using actual words, such as by the therapist's relaxed, peaceful tone, or even a comfortable pause between words, both of which I oftentimes have seen done by Steve and Insoo.

In addition, I wanted some real-life details, such as whether she had a room of her own, so I could tailor my description so that it reflected the realities of her current life. Real-life details are very important. Beyond that, and more important, my choice of words was dictated by wanting to incorporate her exact words and reflect the reality of her current situation as faithfully and respectfully as possible. Inviting a client to answer the miracle question works best if it is conveyed in an appealing, comfortable way, and that is why I wanted her to imagine being comfortable, neither too hot nor too cold, and eventually having the pleasure of sleep while still acknowledging that she had in fact not been sleeping well recently.

Where did you get the idea to put the scale question inside the miracle question?

If she and I had more time, I probably would have simply continued scaling and reached the solution that way. However, we were under a time constraint and she had indicated that she needed to make a decision "soon," so I combined scaling and the miracle question to accelerate the process.

YVONNE: Hmm. Meaning, Paul?

MARGARET: Yeah. Yeah.

Her first answer to the miracle question, "It's not the first thing on my mind," is actually a negative. Some people, especially beginning students of SFBT would likely think this was not a useful answer, but for you it was obviously useful. How so?

For me it was a beautiful opportunity to invite her to go into details of what she would be thinking about instead. "Instead" is a wonderful sort of linguistic doorway that invites clients who have answered with a negation to walk right into a nice description of the solution. In this way, saying he would not be the first thing is a perfect answer, and it indicates that she has made up her mind that she is going to go up on the scale rather than down on the scale.

There is a whole class of what seems to beginners in SFBT or new therapists as "wrong" answers to the miracle question, and the challenge is for the therapist to find a way in each case to respectfully utilize the answer in a way that allows the client to continue with the solution-building process.

For example, the client might say, "After the miracle I wake up and I have won the lottery"; what does the therapist do to get back to a more practical description of a solution?

I respond by saying humorously, "If you do win, will you share it with me?" and then either the client automatically returns to a more practical description of what life would be like when the problem is solved, or at this point, I can comfortably invite him to do so.

Sometimes a client answers the miracle question by saying that "he would be doing something different"; what question do you follow up with there in order to help the client continue in the direction of the solution?

I would say, "Let's suppose, he in fact *did* that, what then would you be doing?"

YVONNE: What might you be thinking of instead?

MARGARET: *[Sighs.]* I think just anything. Maybe something I would do that day.

YVONNE: Like what you would be planning to do that day?

MARGARET: Yeah . . .

YVONNE: Hmm. With friends or on your own or . . . ?

MARGARET: Well, I think I will have to look for work, for example.

YVONNE: Hmm.

MARGARET: And soon, yeah.

YVONNE: So, maybe you might be thinking about possible work?

MARGARET: Yeah.

I am more apt to continue the miracle question and apply it to the scale if I am pressured by time constraints.

YVONNE: Hmm.

MARGARET: I do that now. But, but, now I'm just like so confused. So I think I have to wait.

YVONNE: Mmm-hmm. So you're confused sometimes. But you're doing it now some. You're thinking about it.

MARGARET: Yeah.

YVONNE: That's interesting. So at least you're thinking about it.

MARGARET: But it feels like something's stopping me.

YVONNE: Sure. Yeah. You know. It might not be the time yet. But you're thinking about work.

MARGARET: Yeah.

YVONNE: Sometimes . . . Sometimes first?

MARGARET: No.

YVONNE: When you wake up?

MARGARET: No.

YVONNE: You're thinking about it. So after this miracle or this blessing, maybe you'd be thinking about something else first. It might be plans. It might be what you were doing. What else would be different that you would say, "Ah, this is more of a 7 or an 8"?

Wittgenstein asks: "But how do I know what I would do if . . . ? If I stepped out into the street and found everything completely different from what I was used to, maybe I would just go ahead and join in. So I would behave quite differently than ever before" (LWPP, #200).

MARGARET: Um, I think it would be different also because now they don't know what I'm thinking about. They don't know that I have had this contact with Paul. And, I don't like lying, but I . . . I also feel that I'm lying for them.

YVONNE: Hmm.

MARGARET: Well, I do.

YVONNE: Mmm-hmm.

MARGARET: So . . .

YVONNE: So if you're at a 7, um . . . what would be going on? What would you be doing instead of the lying?

MARGARET: I think it would be easier for me to just talk and be with them. Right now, I'm just like: "Don't ask me anything."

YVONNE: So they'd notice you talking to them more?

You made a shift here from what the client would notice to what Marilyn [the woman in the family] would notice. Why?

Asking a question incorporating the view or reaction of someone with whom the client has a relationship anchors the therapeutic change more concretely in the client's real life, and provides a signpost of progress that she can look at in the future when she in fact does what she is describing and the other person responds. We know that sooner or later she is going to be talking to Marilyn because she is living with her, and she is a woman, and women tend to talk to one another.

MARGARET: Yes.

YVONNE: Just in general.

MARGARET: Yeah. Because I'm sure that Marilyn, the woman in the family, noticed that something is not right.

YVONNE: Because you're so quiet?

MARGARET: I'm not really quiet, but I don't like talking about what I would like to do or what I'm thinking about because then I have to lie even more.

YVONNE: Uh-huh. So she would notice you talking about plans for the future?

Are relational questions like this an integral part of SFBT? Yes. We incorporate these sorts of questions wherever possible in our sessions. Not only does it help the client elaborate the details of the solution, oftentimes it works when the client is unable to find his or her own "voice" in reference to the problem that brings them to therapy, or, more significantly, the goal that they want and need to achieve in order to leave therapy feeling satisfied. There are many clients who are unable to describe what they want to have happen as a result of therapy by thinking solely about what they want or how they personally would know things are better, yet are able to do so very well when asked to describe what others would notice about them that would indicate that things were better.

MARGARET: Yeah.

YVONNE: What's different about the times when you've been able to do that before with her?

In response to this question, the client gives herself good reasons for being honest. This is much more effective than anything the therapist could have said.

MARGARET: Ah, well, I guess when you're honest, it's . . . you're happier and . . .

YVONNE: Hmm. So, happier. How do you feel that? I mean, for you do you feel it in your body, or how do you feel it?

MARGARET: Yeah, I can feel it in my body, too. Right now I'm like . . . in the nights I have this . . . I had a hard time breathing and I'm just nervous and I smoke all the time. And . . .

YVONNE: Mmm-hmm. So you can remember times when the breathing was easy and . . .

MARGARET: Yeah.

YVONNE: You felt . . . you felt happier, more relaxed?

MARGARET: Um, yeah, maybe. But I mean, I just have had this contact with him for like a month or something. So it's not that big of a difference yet.

YVONNE: Hmm. Is that what keeps it a 4? Because it hasn't been going on that long?

MARGARET: Yeah. But, I'm also afraid because it changes so much just from one week to another.

YVONNE: Mmm-hmm.

MARGARET: Like at first, I just phoned him maybe twice a week. Now, I phone him twice a day.

YVONNE: Mmm-hmm. So, if you were at a 7 with this miracle in terms of confidence about whatever your decision is, what else would be different, so that you'd know you were a 7? If you're calling him twice a day at a 4, what would you be doing at a 7?

MARGARET: I don't want to phone him at all.

YVONNE: Really? Would that be a good 7?

MARGARET: Yeah.

YVONNE: It's a pretty big change.

MARGARET: *[Laughs.]* Yeah.

YVONNE: Hmm.

MARGARET: Because I know I can't . . . I can't. I have to do . . . I have to stop everything. I can't like just phone him once a week because then I feel like I'm just losing everything else.

YVONNE: How did you figure that out? From experience or . . . ?

MARGARET: Yeah.

YVONNE: Hmm. So how much would you phone him at a 7?

MARGARET: Well, it would . . . it would be all right for me to phone him once a week if I could handle the situation.

YVONNE: Mmm-hmm. Mmm-hmm.

MARGARET: But, I still want to be sure that it's okay, I have my life here and I won't go back. All right. Right now I think I will (go back).

YVONNE: So, there's something about "I have my life." So in this miracle, you're confident. And part of that confidence is the feeling of "I have my life?"

MARGARET: Yeah.

YVONNE: What will be some signs to you of "I have my life?"

MARGARET: Um. Um. *[Sighs.] [Pauses.]* Maybe I would start to work. I would start to have more friends down here. I also have a place . . .

YVONNE: A house, too?

MARGARET: An apartment in [name of a town]. Where I live like one day a week or so.

YVONNE: You have an apartment?

MARGARET: Yeah.

YVONNE: Would that be part of this, too?

MARGARET: Yeah.

YVONNE: How did you manage to get an apartment? You're young. This is impressive.

MARGARET: No, it's not. Because I had my furniture in [name of town] when I moved from there, and I don't know, what do you call it, social services?

YVONNE: Yeah.

MARGARET: Yeah. They supported me when I said I don't want to have my furniture back there.

YVONNE: So they must have believed in you.

MARGARET: Yeah.

YVONNE: Enough to support you.

MARGARET: Yeah.

YVONNE: Oh. Hmm. I wonder what convinced them?

MARGARET: Um, well, they've known me for a couple of years now.

YVONNE: So they must see something in you.

MARGARET: Yeah, I think so. They're great.

YVONNE: Mmm-hmm. Well, I wonder what they're seeing in you that makes them say "Well, it's worth supporting her with this apartment."

MARGARET: Um, I think many drug addicts are . . . not liking them. And I think they have a hard time helping people.

YVONNE: Mmm-hmm.

MARGARET: But, I've never been like . . . like that.

YVONNE: They saw something different in you?

MARGARET: No, I don't think I'm different. I think since I was a child, I had . . . I think I maybe had a little bit different childhood because I have really great parents. And, if I compare to my friends, I think in one way I had a better time when I was a child. So, I think maybe that gave me something.

YVONNE: Mmm-hmm. And you recognize that, it sounds like.

MARGARET: Mmm-hmm.

YVONNE: So back to the 7.

MARGARET: Mmm-hmm.

YVONNE: So far, let's see, the work . . .

MARGARET: Mmm-hmm.

YVONNE: . . . would be coming in there. You'd be moving toward work?

MARGARET: Yeah.

YVONNE: Moving toward new friends, or old friends?

MARGARET: New friends.

YVONNE: New friends. Okay. In this area?

MARGARET: Yeah.

YVONNE: What about the apartment? How does that fit in?

MARGARET: Well, I think maybe if I spend more time there. Maybe if I can decide a little bit more for myself instead of everybody else deciding what I shall or shall not do.

YVONNE: Hmm.

MARGARET: And if I was able to make good decisions. *[Laughs.]*

YVONNE: So making some good decisions in these other areas?

MARGARET: Mmm-hmm.

YVONNE: Would that give you more confidence toward a 7?

MARGARET: Yeah, I think so.

"But the exception and the rule could not change place without destroying the game . . . 'If exception and rule change place then it just is not the same thing anymore!' But what does that mean? Maybe that our attitude toward the game will then change abruptly. Is it as if after a gradual loading of one side and lightening of the other, there was a non-gradual tipping of the balance?" (RPP1, #145-146).

YVONNE: Hmm. What are some times when you've made good decisions in the past?

MARGARET: Well, I did make the decision to come here and I'm still doing decision to stay here. Do you understand me?

YVONNE: How did you do that? I think I understand. I mean how did you do it? I mean, because that sounds quite significant.

MARGARET: I really do want to live. I really do want to have a good life, a normal life.

YVONNE: Mmm-hmm. Mmm-hmm. Is that part of the 7?

MARGARET: Yeah.

YVONNE: Hmm. Anything else I should be asking you about that might be part of the 7 after this miracle?

MARGARET: *[Laughs.]* No . . . I don't know. Uh, I think also at the point of 7, I'm not so afraid. Now, I'm like afraid for everything. I'm afraid like I will make the wrong decision. I will say the wrong word or . . .

YVONNE: Mmm-hmm. Mmm-hmm. So what would you be feeling and doing instead at the 7 not being afraid? How do you act when you're not afraid?

MARGARET: Um, well, I think I'm laughing a lot and happy.

YVONNE: Hmm . . . So your sense of humor comes back?

MARGARET: Yeah.

YVONNE: Huh. Is that a 7 or is that higher?

MARGARET: No, I think 7 is good enough. *[Laughs.]*

YVONNE: Wow. So laughing. Do you have a pretty good sense of humor?

MARGARET: Yeah, I think so. *[Laughs.]*

YVONNE: Uh-huh. Uh-huh. So is there anything that we should ask Harry?

MARGARET: Um, I don't really know if there's something special to ask him. What do you think?

YVONNE: I trust your instinct, actually.

MARGARET: *[Laughs.]*

YVONNE: It sounds like part of that 7 is maybe trusting your instinct. Shall we see if he wants to ring us with anything?

MARGARET: Yeah.

YVONNE: So you can phone us if you want. *[This is directed toward the team behind the mirror.]*

[Pause.]

HARRY: We were just talking, saying that you don't miss anything. Did you tell me to come in?

YVONNE: We wondered if maybe you had any thoughts or ideas?

HARRY: I think you covered it. I think you sort of laid it out very cleanly: where the dilemma is and what the options are. I think you're very clear. I would have to think about this before adding anything. I don't have any more questions or things that I feel are necessary at this point.

MARGARET: Okay.

YVONNE: Do you want to take a short break and you think about it and I'll think about it a little bit?

MARGARET: *[Laughs.]*

HARRY: Are you okay?

MARGARET: Yeah. Yeah. Good.

YVONNE: You're a very articulate young lady.

MARGARET: Thank you.

YVONNE: How old are you?

MARGARET: 22.

YVONNE: I thought, not from your looks . . . you look very youthful, but just . . . I would have thought you were even a little bit older in terms of maturity.

MARGARET: *[Laughs.]*

YVONNE: Okay. Is there anything else I should have asked?

MARGARET: No. *[Laughs.]* I don't think so.

YVONNE: We'll just take a short break. Do you want anything? Water?

MARGARET: No, I'm fine.

YVONNE: I'll be back in just a few moments.

* * * *[Pause for Break]* * * *

YVONNE: Well, I wrote down a lot of stuff.

MARGARET: Okay.

YVONNE: One of the impressions that everybody had . . . there were several that everybody had. One was that you're a thinker.

MARGARET: Mmm.

YVONNE: And it looked to us like it's useful for you to do that. I mean, that works from what you're saying. I mean, when you think things out, use your own head as you say, it seems to make a difference.

MARGARET: Uh-huh.

YVONNE: From what you described. everybody noticed that, that you're a thinker. Um, you said you've been thinking this over for a while, and it seemed to us, I really feel this way, that there's a good reason. I mean there's a reason you're taking your time with this. Because you want to make the decision that's best for you.

MARGARET: Uh-huh.

YVONNE: And, uh, boy, I just personally had this response . . . of really encouraging you to not go any faster than you are ready to go. To just take it slow. Just like you're doing.

MARGARET: Mmm-hmm.

YVONNE: Because, I don't think how fast you make decisions is what matters. Um, it seems to me that it's more important for you to do what you're doing and really think about all the aspects of this. Um, one person back there pointed out, um . . . there was a lot of head nodding about this . . . everybody agreed. We said, "She is making . . . " you're making, "a very good analysis" of your own situation.

MARGARET: Mmm-hmm.

" 'But the inner is hidden from me'—isn't that just as vague as the concept of 'inner'? (For just consider: the inner after all is sensations + thought + images + mood + intention, and so on)" (LWPP, #959).

YVONNE: And it took some doing, I think. That took some thinking. That's hard work. In talking about that, I felt that in here when I was listening to you: This is not an easy decision. This is a difficult situation because it's going to affect your life. And, I said to myself, "God, this is really a hard decision. It's a shame that someone this young has to make such a difficult decision." And, um, especially because of that, we felt it was so wise of you to not hurry it, to go slow. Take your time with it. Don't decide when you're not ready. Just decide. And, um, they thought that taking it slowly as you are was the most responsible thing you could do.

MARGARET: Okay.

YVONNE: There's another piece of feedback. Um, that it is very important to do as you do. To think about everything so that you have a feeling of confidence that you really are making the right decision. And our thought was that it would be very important to just pay attention to things that would mean moving in the direction . . . you know, work, friends, even interest in work, or something kind of tickles your interest, or the apartment, any signs that would indicate that you moving in the direction of a 5 or a 6 or a 7. Really pay attention to those.

MARGARET: Okay.

"If you observe [pay attention to] your own grief [inner process], which sense to you use to observe it? A particular sense? One that feels grief? Then do you feel it differently when you are observing it? And what is the grief that you are observing, is it one which is there only while it is being observed?" (LWPP, #407).

YVONNE: Because you're on to some of the ways that might be signs. There may be others, too, that will come up. I thought it would be really important to just pay attention to those and to keep doing as you are. In terms of the slowness.

MARGARET: Okay.

YVONNE: And the final thing was: I should ask you if you want to talk to Harry to make an appointment.

MARGARET: *[Laughs.]*

YVONNE: To follow up on . . .

MARGARET: Yeah.

YVONNE: . . . on how this goes. Would you be willing to pay attention to those signs?

MARGARET: Yeah.

YVONNE: Okay.

MARGARET: Yeah.

YVONNE: I get the feeling there's, I'll be curious what you think about this . . . but it seems like there's an ecology to the way you're doing this. There must be a reason you're not rushing this.

MARGARET: Yeah, there is. I think what I did wrong before was . . . I was just living my life from what I felt in my heart.

YVONNE: Mmm-hmm.

MARGARET: And, that was not too good. So now, I'm trying to use my head as well before I make, before I make a decision to do anything.

YVONNE: Yeah. Yeah. Well, from what I understand from the way you describe this, you'd be right. There's some horsepower here [indicating Margaret's head]. I mean there's some stuff there.

MARGARET: *[Laughs.]*

YVONNE: And boy, I think you're absolutely right to . . . to use both.

MARGARET: Yeah.

YVONNE: Okay. Well, I really appreciate meeting you.

MARGARET: Yeah.

YVONNE: And I'll let you talk with Harry. I probably won't get a chance to see you again.

MARGARET: No.

YVONNE: Um, I just want to say I really believe in you. I just have this instinct. And every once in a while I meet a young person and I kind of say to myself afterwards, and I probably wouldn't say it if I was going to see you again. Maybe I'd say it if I ran into you in a year or two. But since I am probably only going to see you once in my lifetime, I'm going to just say: There's something about you. You're one of those young people that . . . you give me hope in the next generation. I just have that feeling. I want you to know that.

MARGARET: Thank you. Thank you for seeing me.

YVONNE: It was a pleasure to meet you. Harry is going to come back.

MARGARET: Okay.

YVONNE: Good luck with this.

MARGARET: Thank you.

YVONNE: I believe you're going to make the right decision for you.

MARGARET: Okay. Yeah. Thanks.

You have created a different linguistic reality for the client through the use of scaling questions, relational questions, and the miracle question, but she is going to leave the session and go back to a life that is very different from this. How do you make the behaviors associated with the solution accessible in her real life?

By answering the relational questions and scaling questions I ask, and answering some of the questions about details, the client constructs an associational and linguistic bridge between her everyday life in the hours, days, and weeks ahead, and the ideas in reference to the solution we talked about in this session. As she goes about her life and does those daily activities and sees those people we incorporated into the questions, she will be continuously reminded of her solution and exceptions.

One could have hoped that after this wonderful session with Yvonne Dolan Margaret would come to her senses, get out of this destructive relationship with Paul, and start building a new life for herself. Well—she did and she didn't. Over the course of a couple of months following the session she started spending more time in her apartment, she developed friendships with more "normal" people, and she got a job in a café. She was clearly building a life of her own in Kayville. She also continued the relationship with Paul but made some interesting shifts in that relationship: She told me she had started to ask questions. "So what do you want to do with your life?" and he would answer "Haven't I done a lot!!!?" and she would go on with "Sure . . . and what do you want to do now?" and he would answer "You'll see . . ." and she wouldn't get more out of him. In the second session after Yvonne's, she said to me: "That is not good enough."

She cancelled the fourth session because she was too busy. Her boss was going away and he was leaving her in charge of the whole business so she simply didn't have the time.

A year after the session with Yvonne she came back with her father and the foster mother. She made it clear that the initiative for this session wasn't hers but theirs. They were concerned about her continuing relationship with Paul and her plans about him eventually moving in with her again. When I (HK) asked her where she was on "the scale," she said that the scale we had used was no longer relevant—she had reached all the goals she had set for herself when she came to me. On a new scale where 10 meant life is exactly the way she wants it and 0 was when she first came, she set herself at 7.

I asked them all what had become better—and what signs there were with Margaret that told them things were moving in the right direction. Father and Lena both talked about a greater attentiveness to other people, a greater capacity to enjoy what she had, and an even greater ability to do what she decided to do.

The problem they saw was what they both called "her fear of losses, which made her get into destructive relationships with men and this was caused by Father's betrayal of her when she was a child." Margaret said she didn't feel betrayed but Father insisted. They tried to explain to me: When Margaret was 10 years old her mother developed a brain tumor that left her incapacitated. The parents were divorced and Margaret was then staying with Father, who developed (or already had) a serious alcohol problem (thus the betrayal). She started cutting herself when she was 12. She developed anorexia in the following years. When she was 16 she started doing drugs and by the time she was 19 she was an experienced heroin addict.

By the end of the session we all agreed that things were moving in the right direction despite all and no further appointment was set. Six months passed. Margaret called and said she was pregnant with Paul and she needed to make a decision about keeping the child or not.

Over the six months that followed we had seven sessions. She had an abortion and for a couple of months she was in very bad shape. She told me about one occasion where she cut herself again—the first time in many years. She had terrible anxiety attacks but at the same time she was able to continue with her normal day-to-day life: working, seeing friends. Paul moved in with her at the beginning of the summer but things were not going well at all between them. Within two months he had hit her when he was drunk and they decided together that this was the end of it and he was moving out. She was terribly anxious when he moved but started pretending that they were still together and that helped her cope with at least some of the anxiety.

She slowly stabilized, and then began to improve. She brought in her closest friend to the second-to-last session and she brought her mother to the last session.

At the time of this writing it's been seven months since I saw her last. On the phone she told me last week that she had moved back to the town where she was born. She is back in school—getting an academic degree at the university. She tells me that she feels really well when she doesn't think about Paul and she is successful with this most of the time. Her studies are going very well and she is very satisfied with being a student.

Chapter 3

The Miracle Question

Based upon our many years of collective "firsthand" experience observing our clients, our colleagues, and (albeit sometimes self-consciously) ourselves "doing" solution-focused brief therapy using scales and miracles, this chapter will explore the multifaceted details, technical subtleties, and paradoxical "simplicity" of the miracle question in the contexts of the client-therapist relationship, problem disappearance, and solution development.

A BRIEF HISTORY OF THE MIRACLE QUESTION

The miracle question came into being by happenstance. Insoo Kim Berg first experimented with this intervention in response to a client, who said in desperation, "Maybe only a miracle will help" (DeJong & Berg, 1998, p. 77). Berg and her colleagues quickly discovered the usefulness of this concept for inviting clients to imagine how life will be once the problem has disappeared. Steve de Shazer (1988) originally worded the miracle question(s) as follows:

> Suppose that one night, while you were asleep, there was a miracle and this problem was solved. How would you know? What would be different? How will your husband know without your saying a word to him about it? (p. 5)

Other solution-focused therapists use similar wording. Peter DeJong and Insoo Kim Berg (1998) recommended the following:

> Now, I want to ask you a strange question. Suppose that while you are sleeping tonight and the entire house is quiet, a miracle happens. The miracle is that the problem which brought you here is solved. However, because you are sleep-

> ing, you don't know that the miracle has happened. So, when you wake up tomorrow morning, what will be different that will tell you a miracle has happened and the problem which brought you here is solved? (pp. 77-78)

Apparently Simple, But Not Necessarily Easy

The words are so simple. It should be easy, right? Watching a master therapist like Insoo Kim Berg ask the miracle question, it does look easy. But upon closer examination, one realizes that despite her relaxed demeanor, and soft, restful tone of voice, she is completely focused on the client every second, fully absorbed and aware of every nuance, every word, careful to not miss any hint about what he or she is wanting from the session, attentive to any and every explicit or implicit reference to struggles, longings, dreams, goals, resources, strengths, relationships, and fragile hopes.

And yet she makes it look easy. This perhaps should not surprise us, as the paradoxical combination of apparent ease and fully absorbed attention is also characteristic of master performers in other fields. Watching the musician Yo-Yo Ma, who is very technically skilled, one often has the impression that he is simply enjoying himself playing the cello, and then it occurs to you that what you are hearing is technically and artistically perfect. He makes it look so easy.

More Than Meets the Eye

To those inexperienced with or uninitiated to the subtleties of therapeutic communication, it would seem that the process of asking the miracle question effectively and then making practical therapeutic use of the clients' responses would be quite a simple proposition. As most people quickly discover, this is usually not the case.

First of all, the interview that leads up to the miracle question requires discipline and self-restraint on the part of the solution-focused therapist. He or she must refrain from interpretations and unsolicited suggestions while remaining attentive to every verbal and nonverbal nuance of the client's unfolding description of the solution.

Furthermore, the miracle question requires an alteration in both the therapist's and the client's everyday way of thinking. And this is a rather rapid paradigmatic shift from the way most people conceptualize and talk about problems both in therapy and everyday life. Let's take a moment here to examine the general construction of the miracle question described earlier in this chapter. Simply, the concept is:

> A miracle happens while you're sleeping—and the miracle makes the problems that brought you here disappear.
>
> But this happens while you're sleeping so you can't know it happened.
>
> How do you and people close to you discover this miracle happened?

The construction is thus that a miracle happens, causing the problems that brought the client into therapy to disappear. However, nobody knows the miracle happened until they begin to see signs of it, and so the client and therapist go on a collaborative search in the client's real, everyday world to discover the signs that indicate the miracle has happened and the problems are gone. Signs of this miracle can only be found in the client's real world, so the miracle question can also be considered the reality question.

THE THERAPIST'S MIND-SET

We think it makes a difference whether or not the therapist assumes that clients have the capacity to create meaningful descriptions of what they want their lives to look like and how they want to be in the world. Asking the miracle question both implies and demands faith in the client's capacity to do this and the question needs to be asked in a manner that communicates this faith.

When asking the miracle question, or teaching the concept in training seminars, we have learned that the way you ask the question is very important, i.e., you have to ask the question as if you really want to hear the answer *and* you believe the client has the ability to give a good answer.

Some therapists are afraid to ask the miracle question because they do not have faith that their clients have the capacity to answer it productively. This results in a sort of catch-22: Faith that clients experiencing serious problems will be able to answer the miracle question can only develop as a result of hearing clients respond beneficially; however, the therapist won't ask questions to invite these responses if he or she doesn't have faith in the clients' capacity to create them. If we believe that a client has the capacity to describe a problem then we must also believe that he or she is capable of describing what "better" than that problem would be.

Over the years in our training programs and workshops, we have heard people ask, "Aren't you afraid that this sort of question might lead people into false hopes or denial? What do you do if a client with AIDS says he won't have AIDS, or a man whose wife left him answers with "She'd be there in the bed with me when I woke up"?

We believe that in most cases people who come to therapy are all too aware of the realities of the conditions they are experiencing, and have the ability to recognize wishful thinking for exactly what it is. On the other hand, starting out by acknowledging what one hopes for that is not going to happen can be a first step toward identifying some useful things that *are* possible to make happen. Steve de Shazer tells a story of a client who lost his left arm in an industrial accident. When asked the miracle question the client answered that he'd wake up with his left arm in place. Steve answered "Sure," and since he didn't know how to go on he waited. A long silence ensued and then the man added: "I guess you mean something that could happen," and Steve nodded. The man then went on to describe how he would get up and make breakfast with only one arm. There was never any talk again about getting the arm back.

It is obvious that many people with serious illnesses and handicaps wish they were well ("he'd wake up with his left arm in place") and there is no danger in them expressing this. When we acknowledge and validate ("Sure"), most people move to a realistic view (". . . I guess you mean something that could happen").

Clients know what's possible and what isn't. They know that talking with us won't give them back their arms, bring back the dead, or cure them or their loved ones of AIDS. Furthermore, it is important to recognize that ultimately the miracle question is not so much about figuring out what would be a "dream come true" miracle for this person or family as it is about discovering, identifying, and replicating the tangible, observable effects of it.

FOUR REASONS FOR ASKING THE MIRACLE QUESTION

One Way to Create Goals for Therapy

Solution-focused brief therapy has its roots in the nonanalytic brief therapy tradition. One thing all brief therapy has in common is that it starts with the end, i.e., trying to figure out how clients will know they have achieved what they wanted from therapy, and knowing when to end. The miracle question is one of the best questions in our repertoire for helping clients describe how they will know therapy is over and one that consistently provides useful descriptions. But it is a difficult question to ask and it is hard work learning how to hold the frame of the miracle in the conversation and continuing to look for the effects of the miracle in the clients' real life. So if this was the only reason to ask the miracle question there are lots of other questions that can do the job almost as well.

The Miracle Question As a Virtual Miracle (or the Miracle Question As an Emotional Experience)

Regularly—not every time the question is asked, but regularly—and more often with the increasing experience of the therapist, clients will behave as if they are experiencing what happens the day after the miracle. Clients will accompany the descriptions with bodily movements as if they were doing and experiencing what they are describing. Sara describes that the morning after the miracle she will go out on the terrace with her tea and sit down in the sun, and as she says this she raises her face toward the sun that is clearly there for her. Victoria's mother shows with gestures, facial expressions, and tears what happens when Victoria becomes "huggy" the morning after the miracle. Anna and her mother stretch their hands toward each other and touch as they describe what will be different between them the morning after the miracle.

The sense I (HK) get whenever this happens is that it is like a rehearsal of the miracle or a virtual experience of the miracle and when it happens I always think "So this is how close it is. These people can simply go home and do it. Wow." It's a humbling experience and one that often inspires awe in clients' possibilities.

It is something that happens very rarely (if ever) when the miracle question is not asked, and it is the strongest reason for asking the miracle question.

Prepares for Exceptions

Among the most useful exceptions and the ones least likely to be ignored are instances of the miracle already happening. When the therapist keeps asking for the details in the miracle picture (the client's preferred future)—"What else will be different after the miracle?"—sooner or later most clients will say things in the general form of ". . . and it happened the other day." This comes as no surprise to us since clients' miracles will always be partly based on hopes for the future and partly on experiences from the past. When time is short and such a comment doesn't happen spontaneously, the therapist can make the transition into this line of thinking by asking, "Do small pieces of this miracle ever happen—even a tiny little piece of it?"

Thus, the miracle question prepares the conversation for exceptions.

Part of Creating a Progressive Story

We have never seen clients spontaneously begin a session telling us that life is great or telling us about all the progress they've made in their lives. Most clients tell what could be called a digressive story—a story about how things are going from bad to worse.

When the miracle question is asked in the way described here, the conversation will move into the parts of the miracle that are already happening and the clients will normally (in most cases) start describing what has become better since they decided to seek help. In all of these sessions, clients will talk about how life is becoming better and some of the clients will even tell us what they are doing that is making their life improve. They are telling us a story about progress and progression. And they will leave the therapy room with a progressive story about what is going on in their life.

HOW TO ASK THE MIRACLE QUESTION

While we occasionally meet therapists who seem to intuitively know how to productively use the miracle question, over the years we have found that most people require some initiation. We have found it useful to follow a few seemingly simple rules:

1. Start by asking something along the lines of "Is it okay if I ask you a strange question?" This serves as a cue to the client that the conversation to follow will be different than usual everyday ones. This is important because answering the miracle question requires a willingness to temporarily suspend everyday assumptions about conversational representations of reality. For many people, the activity of answering appears to elicit a significant shift in their state of consciousness. When we have skipped this introductory question, clients grow restless and sometimes interrupt before we have finished phrasing the question. Wait until the client nods or says "yes" before continuing.
2. Now continue with, "Let's suppose that after we talk here today you leave and you go do whatever you usually do on a day like this. Then as the day goes by you continue doing whatever you usually do. Then you come home, you have dinner, perhaps watch TV, do whatever else you would normally do as the evening goes on." Pick whatever details are appropriate for the client and continue until the client nods. When the question is asked to a whole family it is useful to look at every person in turn and suggest things that seem appropriate for a mother, father, teenager, etc., or do what Steve de Shazer does: Look at the floor or ceiling so as not to indicate who should respond first.
3. When the client has nodded, continue with something like: "Then it gets late, you get tired, you go to bed, and you fall asleep." Wait for a confirmatory nod here so you know the client is following you. Thus far in the question you haven't asked anything. All you've done is invite the client to think about what an ordinary day and evening look like. You want the client to mentally leave the therapy room and imagine the concrete reality of his or her home and the related details of everyday life, because that is where change happens and is noticed.
4. "Then during the night . . . while you're sleeping . . . a miracle happens." It is important to pause here and wait for some kind of reaction: a smile, a lifted eyebrow, or a questioning look. Insoo Kim Berg often looks intently at the client and smiles. Steve de Shazer cautions that it is important to pause here, but not for too long, because in that case clients will pretty regularly say that they don't believe in miracles.*

---

*Sometimes this happens even if the pause is short. I (HK) will often answer "Me neither—but is it okay for you to pretend for a while?"

5. "And not just any miracle. It's a miracle that makes the problems that brought you here today go away . . . just like *that*" (some therapists snap their finger here). Leaving out "the problems that brought you here" is one of the most common mistakes when asking the miracle question and will regularly lead to clients answering with vague, unrealistic goals.
6. "But since the miracle happens while you are sleeping you won't know it happened." At this point, clients typically nod, look thoughtfully at the wall behind the therapist, and generally behave as if they were thinking about this idea.
7. "So . . . you wake up in the morning. During the night a miracle happened. The problems that brought you here are gone, just like that. How do you discover that things are different? What is the very first thing you notice after you wake up?" Over the years we have observed that at this point our clients' bodies typically become very still and their breathing deepens and slows. Their eyes seem to dilate a bit and lose focus. Usually they continue to stare off into space or look down at the floor for a moment or two while they are composing their answer. Oftentimes they even close their eyes for a few seconds. It is important to allow the client time to do this. So make it a point to relax comfortably in your chair, take a nice deep breath, and wait patiently for the answers.

   If there are several people in the room, they will often look at one another and sometimes ask the interviewer who should start.

LISTENING TO THE ANSWERS

Regardless of what words we used, we do not know exactly what question we actually conveyed until we hear how the client answers. It is important to pay close attention because all follow-up questions must be built upon the client's answers. We continue by asking additional questions, listening carefully to the client's response, and then asking further questions based upon that response to further clarify and amplify the details of the client's description.

While every client and therefore every miracle is unique, most of the answers we hear fall more or less into the categories we will explore in this section. While it is always best to incorporate the client's precise words into the questions, we will give general examples of the types of questions we typically ask clients in response to each answer category. Remember that regardless of the words we used in our question, it is not until we hear the client's answer that we can recognize what question the client heard.

There is value in saying that we never know what question we asked before we heard the answer. We believe that such an approach diminishes the risk of us thinking that the client misunderstood us. If we think that we never know what question we asked before we hear the answer, it becomes our responsibility to pay attention to the client's answer as valid and important and this helps us avoid repeating the same question. Thus, clients teach us something about the fit and sequencing of questions every time this happens.

Put differently, if a client answers a question we didn't ask, we know that this is the question we should have asked. Behaving as if we did ask that question helps us learn to be in dialogue. In this way, clients teach us something about how to ask questions and about how to do therapy.

What Does the Client Notice?

Our client (let's call her Sara) wakes up in bed in the morning. During the night a miracle happened and the problems that brought her to therapy are gone. How does Sara first become aware of this? How does she know it happened? What kind of feelings does she wake up with that indicate that something is different, that the problem is gone, what kind of thoughts? Perhaps, most important, what is the first thing that Sara notices that is different, and what exactly does she do that is different as a first sign that the problem is gone? And then, if there is someone else there when Sara awakens, how does that person notice that something is different? How do other people in Sara's life notice it?

As we mentioned earlier, you never know what you asked before you heard the answer and the ensuing questions should be built on the client's answers if there is to be a dialogue.

The "I Don't Know" or Silence Answer

Let's suppose Sara responds to the miracle question with "I don't know." ("I don't know" is one of the most common initial responses to the miracle question.) Our colleague, Dan Gallagher, says that "I don't know" means "Be quiet—I'm thinking" (personal communication, 2000). Over the years, we have noticed that even in situations not involving the miracle question, people commonly preface significant statements with "I don't know . . . ," for example, "I don't know . . . I've been thinking a lot about X (going back to school, leaving a job or relationship, getting married, having a baby, etc.)

We find it especially useful to remain silent for several seconds after the client says "I don't know." We think it is important to allow the person some time to think. We do not repeat the question (unless the client asks us to do so). And we definitely do not comment, nod, or do anything to call attention to ourselves. We have found that it can be helpful to count to six before saying anything else. Doing this without moving, and especially without nodding, is a good exercise in self-discipline on the part of the therapist, and more important, it typically leads to the client starting to develop an answer. This works particularly well if while waiting you lift up your pen and hold it over your pad as if you're waiting for something to write down. If the client hasn't answered in six seconds we thoughtfully say, "It's a difficult question." Then we relax back into our chairs and give the client another six to ten seconds to think.

We cannot overemphasize the importance of the therapist remaining silent during this waiting pause. If you communicate in any other way (verbal or nonverbal), the client will mistakenly start waiting for your next question or statement out of politeness, since he or she will perceive that it is now the therapist's turn to continue. Again, be very careful not to nod or make any sounds that could be interpreted as a response. Otherwise, it can become confusing and awkward for both therapist and client. If you think you didn't say anything additional, but the client thinks you did, the conversation will come to a standstill while the client sits there politely waiting for you to go on and you sit politely waiting for the client to continue the answer.

Of course, once the client moves beyond "I don't know" and starts developing answers, these will naturally vary.

The "Not" Answer

Frequently people begin by describing what they will not feel, will not do, will not think, or how other people will not behave. This is a natural way to think and answer the miracle question. It is often helpful to echo their answer with a little bit of weight on "not" and ask "What else will be different?" Should the client continue with many more descriptions of "not" it becomes useful to ask, "What do you think you will feel (or think or do) instead?" This helps a lot of clients to move on to descriptions of what they will feel, think, or do the morning after the miracle.

We find it useful to think about "feel, think and do" as interrelated parts of the same description. Let's suppose that the client answers the miracle question with how she will feel differently. In this case, we build on this by asking, "So when you are feeling that way, what will you be doing then that you're not doing now?" After listening carefully to the response and acknowledging it, we will follow up by asking "What else?" at least three or four times, each time carefully listening and acknowledging the answers.

We do the same when the client's first answer is "I will think more positive thoughts." In this case, we might ask Sara, "So, when you think more positively, do you have any idea what you will do differently then?" or "What do you suppose you will find yourself doing then?" Since for many clients it is easier to describe how other people will notice the difference, we would also ask, "When you think more positively, how do you suppose your (father/mother/wife/best friend/children) will notice this?" or "What do you suppose your (family member, friend, co-worker) will notice you doing differently that will give them the idea that you're thinking more positive thoughts?"

So let's suppose that after a long and thoughtful silence, Sara answers: "I wouldn't wake up feeling anxious."

The therapist silently wonders to himself: How does one notice this when one wakes up in the morning? What does one feel when "one doesn't feel anxious," or depressed or a huge number of words that we use to communicate with other people about how we feel?

The therapist sits quietly, looks expectantly at Sara, and waits patiently for her to continue. Sara turns toward the window and continues with what now becomes . . .

The Feeling and Thinking Answer

"I'd wake up glad and I'd think, 'Oh, what a wonderful day . . .' I'd look forward to the day."

The therapist echoes: "Wake up glad, looking forward to the day . . . hmm. What else?"

"I don't know" answers Sara and looks at the window again. The therapist is quiet and waits patiently. After a moment, Sara continues: "I'd feel like doing something." We recognize this as the beginning of . . .

The Behavioral Answer

Concrete and detailed behavioral descriptions nicely fulfill Wittgenstein's requirement of an external referent for emotions (See chapters 7 and 8). Therefore, it is probably no surprise that over the years we have usually found behavioral descriptions to be the easiest to incorporate into the therapeutic change process. And it is behavioral descriptions that typically prove to be the most useful for our clients.* Concrete, detailed descriptions of behavior and action constitute a virtual rehearsal of what a person wants to do in his or her life. The more detailed the description, the more vivid and "real" the experience becomes for the client, thereby making it easier and more natural to carry out in real life. The experience of creating a richly detailed behavioral description also allows the client to preview some of the future rewards of the contemplated changes, thereby increasing motivation. Furthermore, if the contemplated behavior involves a much-desired but initially difficult change (such as, for example, leaving a long-term abusive relationship), the positive feelings evoked by this behavioral descriptive process can be an invaluable source of much-needed "courage for the journey."

---

*For a long time, behavioral descriptions seemed to us to be more useful than vague descriptions. We are no longer sure that this is so. With more experience (and through some of the developments of the approach reflected in this book), it becomes easier to work successfully with vague and unclear descriptions using scales.

Concrete behavioral descriptions provide a graceful bridge into interpersonal descriptions of behavior. Let's listen in while the therapist responds to Sara who has said that she will "feel like doing something."

"Feel like doing something . . . How will you notice that?"

This time Sara answers more quickly. "Oh, I'd get up, look at what's in the fridge and prepare a real breakfast. Then I'd wake Andrew . . . No, he's probably already up . . . but, we'd have breakfast together."

Detailed descriptions also seem to help clients "experience" what they are describing. Notice how Sara changed into the present, i.e., "he's probably already up . . ."

This leads the therapist to wonder aloud what Andrew might notice that is different about Sara, which will introduce another category of question.

What Do Other People Notice?

People are not isolated islands floating around in an ocean of solitude. We exist in social contexts. Change isn't change until it's seen and recognized as such in our social contexts. We believe that it is very important to include the client's relationships when co-developing solutions. Sooner or later the client says something that leads us to ask questions about how change will be, and is already, perceived in the client's social contexts. For example, we might now ask Sara,

"What would be the first thing that Andrew notices after the miracle that tells him something is different without you saying a word?"

"What is the first thing Andrew (or colleagues at work, or the children, friends, etc.) would notice you did differently?"

"What would surprise them the most?" (Later in the miracle question when the descriptions are well-anchored in the client's life we might ask, "So suppose all this happens, who would be the least surprised by seeing you do this?")

"What else?"

Many people will begin to answer these questions with descriptions of what people around them would notice is not there anymore.

Let's suppose that Sara answers that "Andrew will see that I'm not irritated (or not depressed or a number of other things that only tell us something about this person's problem). We would answer her in a gentle and friendly tone with something like, "So . . . hmm . . . not depressed . . . hmm . . . so what do you suppose he would see instead of you being depressed?" Or, "What will somehow tell him that you're not depressed (or not as depressed)?"

We focus on creating detailed descriptions of what would indicate to friends and family that there has been a change and the problems are solved. Everything that starts with "not" is essentially regarded as information about the client's problem and not taken into account when thinking about what the client wants. We listen for the presence of emotions, thoughts, and behavior. Often it is helpful to invite the client to imagine what the other person will notice without the client saying a word. For example, we might ask Sara:

"What is the first thing Andrew will notice about you that first morning after the miracle that tells him you are feeling better without you telling him about it?"

Sara thinks for a long time, and looks thoughtfully out the window before answering, "He would notice that I didn't wait for his initiative. He would notice that I would want to do something regardless of what he wanted."

The therapist echoes, questioningly: "He would notice that you took the initiative?"

"Yes . . ." Sara adds: "I don't do anything without him now. I wait for him to say what he wants to do and then I do it regardless of if I want to. Nothing is fun anyway, so it doesn't matter and he notices."*

THERAPIST: So how would that be different after the miracle?

SARA: He would notice that I want to do something. He would see that I am much more joyful and self-confident. I'd suggest something and then I'd do it. I wouldn't care if he was up for it or not.

THERAPIST: How would he notice?

SARA: He would see me smiling, maybe I'd give him a hug spontaneously, and maybe I'd talk about something other than how I feel.

THERAPIST: For instance what?

SARA: It could be anything. A book I read or me telling him I want to see one of my friends. Anything.

This leads us to yet another category of systemic solution-focused questions.

---

*Most therapists are trained in trying to figure out what is wrong with the client and why. Temptation may easily arise at this point to determine why Sara is so "dependent" or why the relationship is like this. If we simply follow intuition, this is where we will go. However, Sara's answer is not an indication that she needs to talk about the problem. This is just the way it is—people tend to answer the miracle question by describing the difference between how it is now and how they want things to be—thus the question that follows.

What Happens Between You?

We exist in interaction with other people. In most cases, we know who we are by how other people respond to us. Descriptions are expanded and given more vividness, richness, and "weight" of meaning by being interpersonal. Recognizing this, at this point in the conversation, we might try to get more details by asking Sara, "How would Andrew react?" "He'd be real glad," she answers, smiling broadly. Let's listen in while the dialogue continues:

THERAPIST: What is the first thing you'd notice with him that would tell you he noticed the difference with you?

SARA: It would take a while. He wouldn't believe it in the morning so he'd probably look at me in a weird way.

THERAPIST: Weird how?

SARA: Like he was wondering. Almost like he was suspicious—but not really, and he wouldn't dare comment on it. *[A broad smile lightens her face and she continues.]* He wouldn't do that for several days. But he'd want us to do what I proposed immediately—a walk on the beach, whatever. He would hook on to my initiative and then he'd look a little bit happier. It's been tough on him—all this time I've been low like this. *[She looks down to the floor, looking sad again.]*

THERAPIST: A little bit happier, hmm . . . How do you see it on him?

SARA: Not so cautious with me, more gladness in his eyes. *[She reflects for a while before continuing.]* It would be the whole way he is acting. Not so guarded and more straight on. He'd take more initiatives to all sorts of things. *[She looks the therapist straight in the eyes and smiles.]*

THERAPIST: Sounds wonderful. *[Sara nods and says "Mmm." Both Sara and the therapist smile.]*

Of course, not everyone responds like Sara. Sometimes the answers become a bit more complex, as in the next category.

The "Things and Other People Will Change" Answer

Occasionally, people begin their response to the miracle question with an unrealistic answer. We think that in most cases this is a result of our not preparing enough before asking the question (an unclear goal), or having made some kind of mistake when phrasing the question. One can feel overwhelmed when this happens. Here are some ideas we have found helpful.

We believe it is valuable for the therapist to remain flexible in wording and rewording the miracle question as needed. For example, in the late 1980s at the Milwaukee Brief Family Therapy Center, a woman answered Steve de Shazer's asking of the miracle question with "If my ex-husband stopped drinking—that would be a miracle." Steve smiled and responded, "Sure." After a short break, the woman continued describing what her ex-husband would do differently toward their children when they visited him. At this point, Steve promptly interjected: "This is a miracle that only hits your house, not his." After this "clarification," she responded with a clear and detailed description, talking about what she would be doing differently toward her kids and how she would eat differently and start losing weight.

We usually respond in a manner similar to Steve's when our clients describe how the world changes for their benefit or when they describe unrealistic events such as becoming rich, winning the lottery, etc. On the other hand, it is possible to go on with questions in which you simply accept the seemingly unrealistic change the client describes and ask what difference it would make for the client. For example, you might say, "Let's suppose you *did* win the lottery . . . What would your wife see you doing, and what would you see her doing that would tell you that that things had gotten better between you?"

We gradually ask a series of questions to clarify what the client would start doing then that he or she is not doing now and how other people would notice it. While this takes patience on the part of the therapist, the answers tend to become progressively more concrete and possible. People generally know what is possible and what isn't.

Perhaps because we have worked in many social service settings involving court-mandated clients, we have frequently heard . . .

The "Social Workers Stop Meddling in My Life" Answer

When clients begin with any variation of this answer, it is important to first respectfully acknowledge how painful it is when social services, the police, or tax authorities meddle in the client's life. The opportunity to productively ask, "So, if the social workers stopped meddling in your life, what difference would it make?" only exists after this is done. You build on the client's answer and this will lead into descriptions of how the client will feel differently and what he or she will do differently.

Another possible direction to go (after acknowledging and validating the client) is: "So, what do you suppose the social workers need to see to get out of your life?"

Seemingly similar to the above answer, but actually not is . . .

The "Family Members Become Different" Answer

"My husband would be more considerate," "My children would obey me," and similar responses constitute a class of answers that we handle in a special way. One important difference is that we don't see these types of answers as necessarily impossible or unrealistic expectations like the above "Things and Other People Will

Change" answer, in which the whole world suddenly is completely transformed for the client's benefit. Instead we look for what's possible, often by simply asking if it is possible and sometimes by first creating more detailed descriptions before asking if it's possible. Let's imagine that Sara referred her Aunt Emma to therapy, and Emma told us that she wanted her son to be more considerate. The conversation might go something like this:

THERAPIST: So what would be the first sign that the miracle happened?

EMMA: He'd get up without telling me to go to hell when I woke him.

THERAPIST: What would happen next?

EMMA: He'd get ready to go to school. Take a shower, get dressed, come down and have breakfast without complaining about it.

THERAPIST: Hmm . . . and what then?

EMMA: Then he'd get his things, his books, his bag, and go to school. *[She pauses, thinks for a moment.]* On time!

THERAPIST: So how would he be different toward you this morning?

EMMA: He'd be friendly. He would smile and talk with me in a normal tone of voice.

THERAPIST: And if he did this, how would you be different toward him that told him that you had noticed?

EMMA: I'd be friendly, too. I would talk with him in a normal tone of voice instead of shouting and yelling and nagging. I get so fed up with him.

THERAPIST: Yes, it sounds real tough on you . . . so . . . how else will you be different toward him?

Gradually the descriptions of life after the miracle lead to questions focusing on whether the different behavior that results (in this case, behaving friendly toward her son) could happen or has already happened at some point in the relationship. If so (this is most often the case), the questions then move in the direction of identifying "when and how" this happens.

As exemplified by Margaret's case, when we encounter this sort of answer to the miracle question, we typically start by accepting the client's description of how the family member becomes different. We then move into asking about how the person who wants the change in his or her family member becomes different as a result of the other person changing. Finally, we ask questions that explore how the interactions change between the people involved.

In short, when working with the "Family Members Become Different" answer, there are usually two phases. The first phase involves asking questions that lead to a description of how the miracle changes the other person. The second phase (which is actually a continuation of the dialogue that began in the first phase) focuses on questions that result in a description of how the relationship between the two people will change, and how this in turn will eventually affect the client who originally wanted the other person to change.

This example also serves to further emphasize one of the key elements of the miracle question that we consider especially crucial: the necessity of developing a richly detailed description of the miracle that is solidly based on the client's real, everyday life. Together with the client and the family we try to create an image of the future in which the problems do not exist and the things that the family wants to have happen do so in such a detailed way that it begins to feel almost as if they have already happened. This is particularly important with families and individuals who have been beaten up by life and are in desperate need of an experience in the therapy room that gives them sufficient courage and hope for the hard work involved in making the solution they envision a concrete reality. For this purpose, we try to create an image of the solution, i.e., life after the miracle, that contains as many concrete details as possible, and we try to "travel" in the miracle picture. We create and we live the miracle with descriptions of emotions, thoughts, behaviors, and interactions with other people. The following case will illustrate this idea.

Karen is in her mid-40s. She had her children late in life and now lives alone with her two teenagers. It seems to the therapist that life hasn't been kind to Karen, and his guess is that she has perhaps had a problem with drinking in the past. She is unemployed, lives on welfare, and was referred to therapy by social services because they are worried about her children. In the beginning of the session, Karen complains about the children's father, who has recently started to harass her again now that he has been released from prison. Let's listen in:

The therapist (HK) has just asked her: "What needs to be different after this session—something small—for you to be able to say that it was a good idea talking with me—despite it not being your idea?" She answers that she would feel calmer and the therapist continues with the miracle question.

KAREN: The kids would stop being disrespectful toward me.

HARRY: So, suppose that happened—how would you be different toward them then?

KAREN: I wouldn't holler so much in the morning. I wouldn't feel so tired and be so irritable.

HARRY: Not so irritable—what else?

KAREN: I wouldn't have to nag them all morning.

HARRY: What would you be doing instead?

KAREN: I wouldn't holler and be so irritated.

HARRY: What would be the first thing that any of the kids would notice, that told them a miracle happened—without words?

KAREN: It'd be Pierre.

HARRY: What would Pierre notice?

KAREN: He would see that I wasn't standing in the doorway and hollering at him to get out of bed. He is impossible in the mornings. He just stays in bed, and it is impossible to get him to go to bed in the evening. He just sits there watching TV.

HARRY: I see . . . so . . . the day after the miracle he would notice that you were not standing there hollering at him . . . hmm . . . what do you think he'd see you do instead?

This question can be seen as an invitation to move into describing the presence of desired behaviors (so far the only thing Karen has described is the absence of problems).

KAREN: I wouldn't be so irritated. *[She stops, thinks for a while, and continues in a somewhat softer voice.]* I'd talk more calmly to him. Maybe I'd go into the room instead of standing at the door yelling. Yeah . . . I'd probably do that. I'd go in and sit down on his bed and I'd say, "Good-morning, Honey. It's time to get up." *[As she says this, a calm smile appears and she stares into space almost as if she is looking right through the therapist.]*

HARRY: Wow! And . . . what do you do next?

KAREN: *[She smiles thoughtfully, thinks for a long time, turns her head to the right and looks down, turns her body a little to the left, and stretches her left arm. It is obvious that she is imagining herself sitting on the side of Pierre's bed with her back toward him and her head turned toward his head.]* I'd pat him gently and wake him up slowly. *[While saying this, she pats gently in the air with her left hand. She looks calmer and the therapist sees her being in Pierre's bedroom waking him up on the morning after the miracle.]*

HARRY: Hmm . . . sounds great . . . so . . . how does he react?

KAREN: I don't know. It's been such a long time since I did it that way. *[She pauses and thinks. The therapist bites his lip. It helps him shut up. After a few seconds she continues.]* He would probably be less aggressive.

HARRY: Hmm . . . and instead of aggressive?

KAREN: He might smile when he wakes up. Perhaps not immediately but at some point he might if I took the time to sit there and talk calmly with him—and then he might even accept a morning hug.

HARRY: Sounds wonderful.

KAREN: *[Nods.]*

HARRY: So tell me . . . suppose that 0 means when the social services decided you should come here, and 10 means it is the day after the miracle—where would you say you're at today?

KAREN: *[Thinks for a long time before answering the question.]* 3. *[She continues spontaneously.]* It's been much worse than it is right now.

Her picture of the effects of the miracle is created out of her hopes for the future and bits and pieces are added from her experiences. It's not a picture that the therapist could have invented for her. It's not a picture built on the therapist's knowledge about how life should be lived. It's her picture and it's developed out of her knowledge and her abilities and we believe that it is also an expression of what she wants. It is a picture that shows her and the therapist the least she can achieve. What she can describe she can also do.

SEVERAL PEOPLE IN THE ROOM

There are advantages with many people in the room. Possibilities are multiplied. When one person stops, the next one continues. When one person describes something, the others are influenced and touched. People listen to one another's ideas about how they will notice a miracle happened and fill in with what they will notice and how they will behave and interact differently.

Young people will almost always surprise their parents with how able they are to articulate what they want and hope for, and with the simplicity of the things they want.

Parents will often surprise their teenagers by being clear about how they want to behave differently toward their children and by being clear about what they want to see happening. Many of the children and teenagers we see are not accustomed to their parents being clear about what they want to see. They are used to hearing what the parents and other adults don't want to see.

Families generally come to therapy with huge differences of opinion regarding what the problem is and who is to blame for it. It's always touching to see these differences lose importance as the family explores the miracle together.

With families, it is generally easier to keep the miracle picture in the family's real-life situation. Questions such as "Who will notice first?" and inquiries about where, when, and how the different people in the room will discover the effects of the miracle all contribute to making the miracle picture anchored in the small activities of daily living.

Mother brings Victoria, age 15, to therapy. When asked who's idea it was to come and see the therapist (Harry Korman), Victoria immediately answers: "Mother's." Mother adds that it was the school's idea, so Harry asks Victoria what she thinks the school and Mother need to see happen as a result of talking with him for them to be able to say it was a good idea sending Victoria to therapy.

Victoria answers: "That it will be better in school and better with my friends after school."

Harry echoes this and asks, "And what do you want?" Victoria answers that she doesn't want to go to school and the problem with her friends is already solved since she stopped seeing them. Mother listens attentively while Harry and Victoria talk about the changes Victoria made and why she made these changes. At this point in the interview, Harry thinks that Victoria doesn't want to go to school and that this is not a problem for her. The problem with her friends that Mother and the school are worried about is solved, so Victoria believes she has no problem.

So Harry asks what could be a slight change that would tell Victoria that it wasn't a complete waste of time coming in to see him despite it not being her idea to come, and after a thoughtful pause Victoria answers: "I'd get the strength to do things."*

Harry echoes: "Get the strength to do things," and continues, "So do you have any idea how you would notice, today or tomorrow, if you got the strength to do things? In what area of your life do you think you would notice it first?"

Victoria looks thoughtful, her eyes wander about the room, and she then says, "It would be about school, I think."

HARRY: About school, hmm. So would you notice it in school or at home?

VICTORIA: I think I'd notice it in school.

HARRY: You'd notice it in school, not at home?

VICTORIA: No.

HARRY: First when you are in school?

VICTORIA: Yes.

HARRY: So do you have any idea what you would do differently there if you had the strength?

VICTORIA: I'd go to my classes.

HARRY: *[Laughs at the obviousness of it.]* You would go to your classes, so it would be a very obvious difference if you felt the strength? *[Mother smiles broadly and so does Victoria, casting a sideways glance at her mother.]*

VICTORIA: Yes.

HARRY: Okay. So if you went to classes and felt the strength, would there be more things that would be different? Would Mom notice any difference at home; would your family notice any difference?

VICTORIA: I think I'd be happier.

HARRY: Happier?

VICTORIA: And nicer.

HARRY: Nicer too?

---

*It's common for teenagers to "deny" problems. In a family session this is no hindrance to asking the child if he or she wants something to be different. Many teenagers will answer with "getting adults off my back" and sometimes, as in the present case, feeling something different.

VICTORIA: Yes, I can be pretty foulmouthed.
HARRY: And you don't want that either?
VICTORIA: No.
HARRY: Okay, so, happier and nicer and everybody would notice that?
VICTORIA: Yes, I think so.
HARRY: Okay, okay, so can I ask your Mom now?

Harry asks Mother what she hopes for and Mother talks about "opening up, finding new ways, and she would know this was happening because then Victoria would stop lying." She then tells the story of the almost three years of unsuccessful attempts with child psychiatry, social workers, assistance in school, etc. to help Victoria with her problems.

Harry returns to "opening up" and asks how Mother would know when Victoria stopped lying, and Mother says she will know. Victoria acknowledges with a broad smile that Mother is right about this; Mother can tell when Victoria is telling the truth and when she is not.

HARRY: So—if Victoria starts telling the truth, how would your mother become different toward you then?

VICTORIA: She wouldn't look so sour.

HARRY: And how would you be different toward your mother then? *[Both mother and daughter laugh heartily at this question.]*

VICTORIA: I don't know.

HARRY: Okay, let's come back to that. *[Pauses.]* It sounds to me like the two of you want things that are clearly in the same direction. *[They both nod after a quick look at each other. It's 14 minutes into the session and Harry asks the miracle question.]* So, a very strange question that takes lots of imagination. Is that okay? *[Victoria answers "Yes" and Mother nods.]* Suppose we talk here today and it goes the way it goes. We don't know how it goes. *[Victoria answers "No" and Mother shakes her head.]* And after this session, you leave, you do the things you normally do on a day like this. I don't know what that is. *[Turns directly to Victoria.]* Maybe you go to school, maybe you don't."

VICTORIA: I go to school.

HARRY: You go to school, and *[turns to Mother]* I suppose you go to work.

MOTHER: Yes.

HARRY: So, the day goes by as usual. Then afternoon comes and eventually you get home. *[Turns toward Victoria.]* Maybe when you're supposed to, maybe not. Maybe you go hang out with your friends, I don't know. Maybe eat. Do your homework or don't do your homework. *[Victoria smiles, shakes her head, and mimes a clear "No."]* And eventually it gets late, you get tired, you go to bed, and you fall asleep. *[Pauses and looks attentively at both.]*

HARRY: And then during the night while everybody is sleeping, when it's the most dark, quiet, and comfortable, a miracle happens. *[Mother smiles broadly while Victoria looks attentively at Harry.]*

HARRY: But it's not just any miracle. It's a miracle that makes the problems that brought you here today disappear, just like that. *[Snaps his fingers and both Mother and Victoria nod quietly.]*

HARRY: But this happens when you are asleep, so no one knows it happened. Not you, not you, no one knows. So you wake up in the morning. How do you notice, how do you discover, "Wow, something is different"? *[Victoria looks at her mother and says, "Yes." Mother is gazing off into the distance.]*

HARRY: What is the first difference? What do you *[to Victoria]* notice? What do you *[to mother]* notice? *[Victoria looks at her mother who slowly and calmly answers.]*

MOTHER: Calm.

HARRY: *[Looks at Mother.]* Say something more about that.

MOTHER: Mmm, Victoria would be cuddly.

HARRY: Victoria would be cuddly. That would be a miracle?

MOTHER: Yes.

HARRY: *[Smiles broadly and laughs.]* Hmm. So where and when would you first notice she was cuddly?

MOTHER: She would come to me immediately.

HARRY: When she got up?

MOTHER: Yes.

HARRY: Who wakes her up? Does she get up by herself?

MOTHER: No, I wake her up every morning.

HARRY: So, would she get up and hug you right there, immediately?

MOTHER: Yes, or pull me down into the bed. *[Mother shows with her arms how Victoria pulls Mother down toward her.]*

HARRY: Okay. I see. *[Turns to Victoria.]* So, suppose you did that. How would she *[nodding toward Mother]* react?

VICTORIA: Well, she would probably be happy.

HARRY: Would you see it on her face?

VICTORIA: Yes.

HARRY: And what would she do then?

VICTORIA: Smile. *[Laughs and smiles happily and the therapist nods vigorously.]*

MOTHER: I would never let go again. *[Tears in her eyes.]*

HARRY: Okay . . . Wow . . . What would happen next? What happens next, this morning?" *[Mother and daughter are looking at each other now, both smiling.]*

MOTHER: Then Victoria would go and get herself together.

HARRY: Get herself together.

MOTHER: Shower, put on some makeup. Get her things, prepare for school.

VICTORIA: *[Nods.]* Hmm.

HARRY: That would be a miracle if she did that.

MOTHER: Yes it would. *[Both Victoria and Mother nod to Harry. Harry turns to Victoria.]*

HARRY: What would be the first thing you noticed?

VICTORIA: I don't know. *[Pauses; her gaze wanders off.]* Wow, school!

HARRY: *[Raises his eyebrows and echoes]* Wow, school, wow, school! *[Mother laughs and Victoria smiles broadly.]*

HARRY: *[Writes and nods.]* Yes . . . that would be a miracle. So if you felt like that, would you notice it before you opened your eyes or after?

VICTORIA: When I woke up.

HARRY: Wow, school! *[Adds tentatively]* Enthusiasm?

VICTORIA: Mmm.

HARRY: Mmm, Mmm, so if you woke up with this enthusiasm, what else would be different? Would it be easier for you to get up?

VICTORIA: I would fly out of bed.

HARRY: And then?

VICTORIA: I'd run to school. *[All three burst out laughing.]*

HARRY: What would they notice at home? If you didn't tell them. Without words?

VICTORIA: Happier, more positive.

HARRY: Happier, more positive. Okay, okay . . . So if I had a video film of you the day after the miracle and one from the day before, with no sound, would I see the difference?

VICTORIA: Yes.

HARRY: How? What would I see?

VICTORIA: The day before?

HARRY: The day after, what would be there?

VICTORIA: The day after the miracle?

HARRY: Yes.

VICTORIA: I would be more . . . I would be smiling, normally I don't.

HARRY: Mmm, and I would see that on the movie. It would be that obvious, I'd see it on the movie?

VICTORIA: Yes.

HARRY: And how would you be different toward Mom? Is Dad there, too?

VICTORIA: Yes.

HARRY: Is he also at home in the morning?

VICTORIA: Sometimes.

HARRY: What would I see you do on the film?

VICTORIA: Hug Dad. *[Mother is listening attentively. She smiles when Victoria says this. Harry sounds surprised.]*

HARRY: Hug Dad. Okay, wow, would he be surprised?

VICTORIA: Yes. *[Both she and her mother nod.]*

MOTHER: He'd faint.

HARRY: He'd faint? *[Sounds even more surprised.]*

MOTHER: *[Happily]* Yes.

HARRY: *[Turns to Victoria.]* Is that true, would he faint?

VICTORIA: Yes, I don't know. *[She laughs and so does Harry and there is a short pause before he continues.]*

HARRY: So this sounds like a very, very, very different start of the day.

VICTORIA: Mmm.

HARRY: What difference would it make in school. Would you be different there?

VICTORIA: Happy, positive, yeah . . . *[Her voice becomes hesitant. She looks uncertain, glances at her mother. Harry continues.]*

HARRY: Who would notice it first?

VICTORIA: Friends. *[Her voice is confident again.]*

HARRY: Do you have a close friend who would be very surprised and see the difference or are there many who would see it?

VICTORIA: Yeah, I think there'd be many.

HARRY: Many would see the difference. So how would they describe the difference? How would they say you were different? What would you do in school then that you don't do now?

VICTORIA: Be nice to others.

HARRY: Be nice to others, wow! So can you give me an example of what that means?

VICTORIA: Help others, don't be so foulmouthed with them.

HARRY: Nice to others, helpful, better language. The teachers, what would they see?

VICTORIA: They would probably faint as well. *[She smiles and looks at Mother, who smiles too.]*

HARRY: They would faint as well. *[Sounds very surprised.]* You mean there would be a great difference in your behavior toward them as well?

VICTORIA: At least I would go to my classes.

HARRY: *[Laughs.]* If you went to classes?

MOTHER: They would think they had a new pupil in the class.

HARRY: If you went to classes, wow. *[Takes notes, nods to himself.]* I'm sorry, Victoria, I'm completely confused. It sounds to me like these are things you want.

VICTORIA: Mmm.

HARRY: Did I get this right? This is how you want to feel and the way you want to be?

VICTORIA: *[Almost whispers.]* Yes.

HARRY: What would surprise your friends the most? What would surprise your environment the most the day after the miracle?

VICTORIA: If I was calm and quiet.

HARRY: Do you mean in school?

VICTORIA: Yes.

HARRY: Would you notice in people around you if they were surprised?

VICTORIA: Yes, they would be nice back.

HARRY: Nice back. That is a difference you would notice as well?

VICTORIA: Mmm.

There is a long silence while Harry looks as if he's thinking. He then says, "Another strange question. If 10 stands for all these things happening, it's the day after the miracle, and 0 is when Mother called and made the appointment here three weeks ago—where would you say you're at on that scale?"

This brings us to the next chapter, in which we will offer many possibilities for making use of the client's answer to questions about the miracle scale.

Chapter 4

The Miracle Scale

As discussed in the previous chapter, once we have succeeded in developing a description of the miracle question, we further expand the dialogue around the miracle by using the miracle scale. We typically introduce the miracle scale with a question that sounds something like the following:

"So, on a scale from 0 to 10—where 0 means when you decided to seek help and 10 means the day after the miracle—where would you say you're at today?" Steve de Shazer argues for defining 0 as when the client decided to seek help, and not when things were at their worst. There are a number of reasons for this. If 0 is when the client decided that he or she wanted help and the client answers 0, you can ask "So what have you done that prevented things from getting worse?" or "How come it hasn't gotten worse?" These questions are possible if 0 is defined as when things were at their worst.

Another argument is that if you define 0 as the worst, this point could be 14 years ago when this or that happened, and with such long time intervals it becomes difficult to create meaningful descriptions of what has become better and how this was achieved. It is important to understand that the greatest value of the miracle scale—as of other scales—is to open up the possibility for a dialogue around differences.

It's possible to move from the "miracle question" to its scale rather quickly and there are advantages to this.* The scale makes it possible to highlight and describe what has already become better and what and how the client did to achieve this. The scale also transforms the miracle from an endpoint to a series of steps—a process whereby each step contains thoughts, emotions, behaviors, and interactions in different areas of the client's life and reality.

*Moving from the miracle question to the scale is not a very good metaphor since the scale is actually a part of the miracle question.

When Can You Set the Miracle on a Scale?

The miracle question explores the client's ideas about the desired tomorrow, sometimes moving into next week or next month. Many clients will spontaneously start telling about parts of the miracle that happened one of the last few days. Listen to what verb forms the client is using. It is common for the client to start talking about "... then I will do ..." After some time the conversation moves into the present tense: "... when I do that he reacts by ..." Many clients will then move on to past tense: "We had a day like that last Tuesday" or "I have started using my head already sometimes ..." The scale thus becomes a logical way to clarify what aspects of the miracle are already happening.

Insoo Kim Berg often introduces the scale after having asked, "When was the last time parts of the miracle happened—even a little tiny bit?" She then listens to the answer, echoes and acknowledges, and then asks "So—if 10 means the day after the miracle ..."

Steve de Shazer once said that he introduces this scale when he can "see the miracle." He looks at the ceiling and uses the client's descriptions. When he has the sense that he can see a picture that is built on the concrete stuff the client has described he says: "So—on a scale ..."

What's the Difference?

It is very unusual in our experience for clients to answer 0 on this scale* when the emotions that will accompany the miracle have been experienced in the conversation. The answer we typically hear is 3, but it is not uncommon for people to answer 5 or higher. The absolute number is not important. What matters is to talk about the difference between 0 and where the client puts himself right now.

So if the client answers 3, we ask: "Hmm ... So what is it that tells you that you're at 3 and not at 0?"

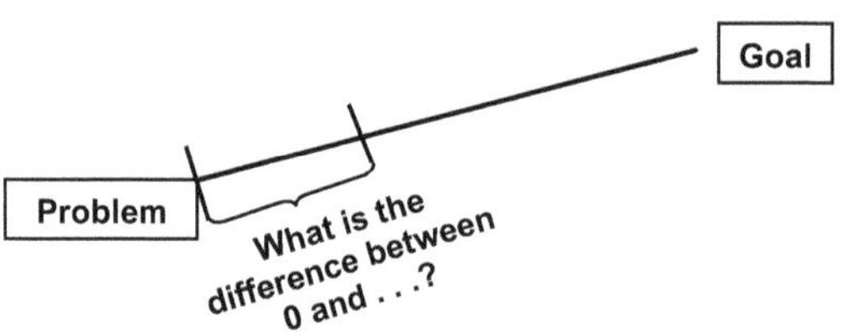

We listen carefully to the answer, we echo, and we summarize. We ask for examples if the client is not providing us with any spontaneously. We try to create concrete descriptions including thoughts, emotions, behaviors, and interactions. Sometimes we ask already here: "How did you make that happen?" or "What did you do that made that happen?" We almost always continue with "What else tells you that you're at 3?"

*It seems to us that the more experienced the interviewer, the rarer it is that clients answer 0.

Remember the enormous difference between this question and questions that have to do with how things were at 0. Clients will sometimes (actually quite often) answer as if we had asked what went on when things were at 0 (maybe because that is the question most nonsolution-focused therapists would ask). It's helpful when we interrupt and ask: "That sounds like when things were at 0?" and when the client has nodded to this we repeat: "So what happens at 3 that doesn't happen at 0?"

The "what else" question is repeated many times so that the client can describe as many examples as possible of what has already gotten better. This question also helps us slow down, further acknowledge, and thereby amplify the things that are already better. This process is like building an effective springboard. The more substance there is below, the more springiness there is. Detailed descriptions help us feel more respect for the clients' competence and abilities and help us get more confident in our knowledge that clients know all they need to know and have all the skills they need to solve their problems.

What Would Other People Say?

"If I asked your boyfriend, where would he say you're at on this scale where 10 is the day after the miracle?" Most clients have clear ideas about what family members and friends think and feel about their situation. The question is of course followed up with questions about what the client thinks that person sees that makes him or her put the client there. When the "other" people are in the room—which is often the case—they are of course asked directly. Interesting and useful differences will often emerge and lead to further questions. "What is it you know about yourself that your mother doesn't know yet?" or "What do you think your mother sees in you that makes her put the number higher than you do yourself?"

How Did You Do It?

It's important in this phase of the conversation to ask questions about "how" the client made things improve. What did the client do and how did he or she manage to do it? We may have to ask this question a number of times and often without getting any clear answers.

Many clients have difficulties describing what they did to make things better. It is therefore important to be persistent even if, and oftentimes particularly if, the client seems to be struggling a bit at first in formulating an answer. The question implies that the client did something valuable; things don't get better without a reason. Therefore, someone must have done something that was helpful. When clients regularly

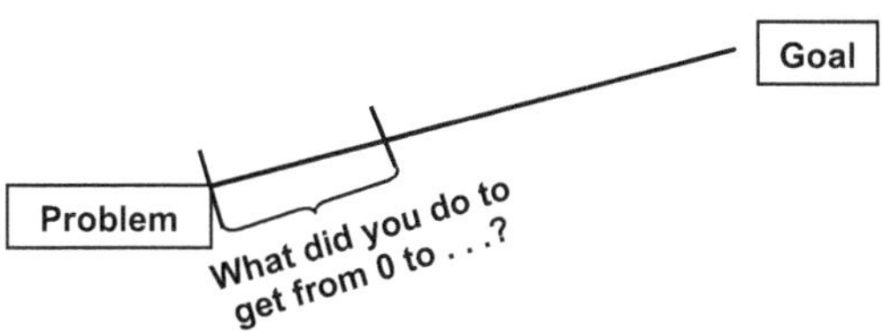

can't figure out what they did that was helpful, we suggest to them that it could be useful to keep doing whatever they are doing and recommend that they pay attention to whatever they and/or other people are doing that is helpful.

It is important to be curious, but it is also important to *only* be curious, that is, to remain neutral. It's easy to fall into the trap of trying to convince the client that he or she did something that made a difference. The risk of this is that the therapist becomes more optimistic than the client. We agree wholeheartedly with our colleague Brian Cade (1997) who said that it is important to never be more enthusiastic about change than your clients, because if you are, you become like their mother and they already have one. It is impossible not to touch on people's resources and competencies when you focus on what people have done that made things better.

Resources and Competence

When we are curious about what clients notice that is different and express this curiosity by repeatedly asking "What else?" clients respond by creating an increasingly detailed description of what is already happening in their lives that they want to have happen. A stance of appreciative curiosity is invaluable for deepening the unfolding description of the solution.

It's helpful to remember the moments when the client and therapist discuss the details of everyday life and to understand the very small things that make a difference to this client. It's then that the therapist understands what the client wants as well as the client's problem. It is then that the therapist may be deeply impressed by how the client has succeeded in doing something that the therapist viewed as banal only a few minutes ago. This is helpful for developing and maintaining respect for client and family resourcefulness. The therapist can then move on to exploring the differences identified with moving up on the scale.

What Is One Step Higher?

The natural question to ask is: "What do you need to do to get one step higher?" We have observed this again and again in therapy and supervision, training exercises, workshop role plays, and supervision. Once, a young man I (HK) was seeing answered this question with "That's your job, that's why I am here, and do you really believe that I would be sitting here if I knew the answer to that question!!!"

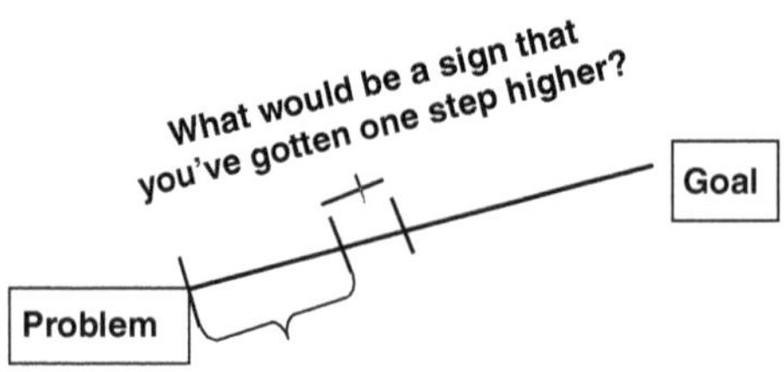

I apologized and asked him if I could try another question and he nodded so I asked: "How will you know that you've gotten one step higher?" He smiled and said, "You're right. That's a question that only I can answer."

When we ask clients how they will notice that they are one step closer to their miracle, it's not possible for them to say that we should know that. It's only the client who can know what would be a sign of progress for him or her. This is an important difference between the two questions. It doesn't matter that a lot of clients will answer with what they need to do to get one step higher when we ask them how they will notice when they've gotten one step higher. Responding with what they need to do implies that they should do something—it's none of our business if they do it or not.

In a discussion with Steve de Shazer (February 2002), Steve observed that a lot of people with drug and alcohol problems know what they need to do for things to become better. With these people the question "What do you need to do?" fits and they can answer it with useful answers.

The Client Answers: "I Don't Know"

As discussed earlier in this chapter, when we believe in our heart that clients ultimately know what they want, even if they don't yet recognize that they possess this knowledge, we are able to remain silent, behaving as if the client has actually said "I don't know yet—give me some time to think," maybe lifting our pens to paper and just waiting without nodding or speaking. Sometimes this can be hard to learn, however. We have found it useful to look at tapes and observe what happens when the therapist doesn't wait. In such cases, it quickly becomes apparent how very easy it is to inadvertently "steal the client's voice."

The Client Answers with the 10

When we've asked, "What would be a sign that you've gotten one step higher?" many clients answer with descriptions of what would be 10 on the scale. This is so common that we have gotten into the habit of responding: "That sounds like a 10?" or "Wouldn't that be 10?" or "That sounds much bigger than 3?" Our clients typically respond with "Yes, it is," and we then move on to ask, "So . . . what would be a tiny little sign?" or "What would be the tiniest little thing that was different that would tell you it was one step higher?"

Because it is oftentimes easier for people to see themselves through another person's eyes, another useful question with the miracle scale is often: "What would be the smallest thing that your children would notice that would make them think it's one step higher?"

It's easier to describe big steps than small ones. The risk with big steps is that they become too difficult or even impossible, thus increasing a feeling of desperation, so we work hard to get the client to describe small steps. After the client has finally succeeded in identifying a relatively small step, we say: "Great! Now what would be something even smaller?" We may repeat this process several times within the same session so the client can identify steps that are ultimately achievable given the realities of his or her life. We strive to ask questions that result in clients identifying a list of those practical, effective, and achievable things that constitute the solutions they desire. Follow-up questions focusing on how other people in the client's life will notice "one step higher" further clarify and refine the description to reflect the realities of the client's everyday life, thus making the goal achievable.

In the event that the client insists that what he or she has described is one step higher and absolutely not more, we accept and acknowledge that. We then ask for details regarding what would subsequently be 2 and 3 steps higher. Sometimes we will go through all the steps up to 10, creating a ladder of how progress will be noticed by the client and his or her social network. (Sometimes, during the session, I [YD] make it a point to note the steps vertically on a piece of paper as per the client's description, and the result is a diagram that visually resembles a ladder as well. At the end of the session, I offer the client the diagram I made. Oftentimes clients tell me that this helps them remember the steps they identified and the goals they set for themselves in our session.)

The Client Answers with "0"

In our workshops, supervision, and training seminars, we are often asked, "So, what do I do if the client answers 0?" If you have defined 0 as "when the client decided that he or she wanted help," you can ask what the client has done that prevented things from getting worse. In the ensuing conversation the client will sometimes tell you that things stopped deteriorating after he or she decided to seek help. Time can then be spent figuring what the client did that was helpful.

You can also ask, for example, questions such as how the client managed to get to your office (or out of bed), or how he has managed to not kill himself, or, if you're talking to a mother, how she manages to cook for her children. All questions about coping can be useful in this situation.

Occasionally, the client is in so much distress that it is seems impossible to create a sense that things are moving in the right direction, or even that things have stopped moving in the wrong direction. We then set up a "hope scale": "If 10 means that you have all the hope in the world that things will get better in the future and 0 means no hope at all, where are you on that scale?"

> Fifteen-year old Rita was at 0 on the miracle scale, and when asked the hope scale she answered 0. The therapist (Harry Korman) responded, "But that's terrible," and Rita nodded. Some seconds passed before Harry continued, "No hope. But—what are you doing here?"* She looked momentarily confused and then answered, "I have to try!" When Harry asked her why she had to try,

---

*Without hope, you don't seek help.

she said that it was because she had no alternative; the only other option was to kill herself, and she didn't want that, and besides it was forbidden by her religion, and "if I try, maybe I'll get some hope." Harry asked her what else made her want to try and after several more answers he asked her how important it was for her to try on a scale where 10 stood for the most important of all. She answered 100. He then asked her how much effort she was prepared to put into it and she answered "One million."

You Never Know What You Asked—Again

Victoria put herself at 5 on a scale where 10 means the day after the miracle, while Mother put her at 3. Victoria believed that her father and the school would put her at the same as Mother. Harry asked her what was better that made her put it at 5 and she answered, "I am calmer and I'm nicer to the people around me. I'm not the big tough one anymore." Harry answered, "Wow—and what else is better?" and she described things about school attendance that were clearly better. Mother clearly agreed with the changes Victoria described and the therapist moved on to "So—how did you get yourself to do this?"*

Victoria answered, "When I started seeing Christine, at first I didn't go to any classes . . . Well, first I had my mentor Tom and I went to classes because he went with me and that was much more fun. When he left school, I skipped classes again. Then with Christine I started getting back into class and the last semester I went to all classes. And now that she has left I'm back to the same thing again."

She talked about what Tom and Christine did some time ago that was helpful so she seemed to be answering the question, "What did other people do that was helpful?" So Harry moved on:

HARRY: Mmm, right . . . and how did you get started again, these last three weeks?

VICTORIA: Mom, and my teacher.

Again she answered with what other people did rather than with what she did herself. There is nothing wrong with that information; it can be useful, so the therapist decided to follow her:

HARRY: What did they do that was helpful?

VICTORIA: My teacher tried to get me back into classes.

HARRY: How?

VICTORIA: Making it more fun.

*It is self-evident that if she can describe what she did that made a difference and how she did it, then she could do it again if she chose to.

HARRY: And what has Mom done that's been the most helpful?

VICTORIA: She nags.

HARRY: She doesn't stop nagging. And what has Dad done?

VICTORIA: He nags.

HARRY: Have you got any friend who's been helpful?

VICTORIA: In physical education I have Minnie, who always says, "Come on now—let's go to the PE!"

HARRY: And that's helpful?

VICTORIA: Yes, that helps and I go to language classes too.

HARRY: Does it work better there?

VICTORIA: Yes.

HARRY: How come?

Harry and Victoria and her mother continued exploring what everyone else had done for a couple of minutes and then Harry returned to:

HARRY: So—that's what everybody else has done . . . So—what is the most important thing you have done yourself that's made a difference? That has gotten you from 0 to 5?

VICTORIA: I tried to change myself.

HARRY: Say something more about that.

VICTORIA: Thinking that I have to make it.

HARRY: Thinking that you have to make it, why do you think that, why is that important?

VICTORIA: So I don't have to listen to all the nagging.

The therapist and mother burst out laughing. Victoria laughs too. Well, it sure is a good reason, but are there more reasons?

HARRY: What else? Do have anything else to win? Do you want to make something out of it? Do you have any plans?"

What is different, why did the client make the change, how did the client make the change, who was helpful, and what are the effects of the change? Answers to any and all of these questions contain useful information. Clients will often describe why they made changes when the therapist asks what is different and will frequently answer with "what is different" when the therapist asks "How did you do that?" Clients will sometimes spontaneously tell the therapist why they decided to make a certain change. Once again, it is important to listen to the client's answer so you know what question you asked.

The Miracle Question and the Following Sessions

Typically the therapist will start the session by asking, "What's better?" and after eliciting some details he or she will ask where the client puts himself or herself on the scale. Some therapists will start the session with the scale and some therapists will start the session saying something such as: "Things go up and down; sometimes it's a bit better, then it's worse, then it goes up again. So, what is the highest and lowest you've been on the scale since we met last, with 10 standing for the day after the miracle?" The client answers with highest and lowest and the therapist then asks what was different when the client was higher on the scale and how the client made it happen. The therapist will also normally ask where best friend, wife, children, etc. would put the client on the scale and what the client thinks they have seen that makes them put him or her there.

Most often clients will be able to describe a number of things that are better in different areas of their life, how they felt better, what they did that was a sign or expression of "better," and how other people were different toward them then. The therapist can ask if these things are new, and will usually ask for the client's explanation about how these changes happened (Who did what that was helpful?). Sometimes clients will be able to describe what they did that made a difference and how, and sometimes clients will respond like Victoria did while explaining how she got herself to go to school every day after the first session: "I have no idea. I have just gone nuts."

A rather typical exchange in the beginning of a second session will be the following:

HARRY: Ten days since last time. So—what's been better?

VICTORIA: "I don't know. *[Thinks for a while before continuing.]* I think I'm calmer; I don't talk as much.

HARRY: Don't talk as much in a positive way?

VICTORIA: Yes, I'm calmer.

HARRY: You're calmer.* In what kind of situations do you notice that you're calmer?

VICTORIA: At school, I go to my classes and I sit quietly and work.

HARRY: Is that a calm you feel inside or is it because you are more quiet or both?

VICTORIA: I think it's both.

HARRY: Both, so when you say talk less is it in general or just less annoying?

---

*Harry remembers that in the first session Victoria said that what would surprise her friends and teachers most would be if she was calm.

VICTORIA: Less annoying.

HARRY: That's the difference. Would your teachers say you were different?

VICTORIA: My homeroom teacher would say so.

HARRY: So if I asked your homeroom teacher—is it a she or he?

VICTORIA: It's a she.

HARRY: What would she say is the biggest, most important difference?

VICTORIA: Since I usually talk a lot, it would be that I am more quiet.

HARRY: Quieter . . . Would she say you're more involved in your schoolwork?

VICTORIA: Yes she would—'cause I'm more quiet and I work.

HARRY: How did you do this?

VICTORIA: I have no idea. I've just gone nuts.

HARRY: You've just gone nuts—so "how" is a big question mark.

VICTORIA: Yes.

HARRY: You don't know how it happened?

VICTORIA: No.

HARRY: Is it a difference that affects you? Do you feel better, worse?

VICTORIA: I feel better.

HARRY: You feel better. Good. So if 10 is the day after the miracle and 0 is . . . , we did talk about the miracle when you were here? Where would you put yourself on that scale today?

VICTORIA: 6-7.

HARRY: 6-7—so a couple of steps better than last time. So—what else is better?

The therapist will generally spend a lot of time asking questions about what is better, what other people see that's been better, how the client knows that other people noticed the difference, and what anyone (including the client) did that was helpful.

Regardless of whether the client is able to describe how the difference came about, the therapist will regularly ask how confident the client is on a scale that he or she can maintain the changes or continue up on the scale. The client's answer to this question will generally initiate a dialogue about what makes the client more confident than 0 that he or she can do it. Sometimes the conversation at this point will turn entirely toward how the client will notice that he or she is more confident and sometimes the conversation will be about signs of further improvement.

It seems useful to think of the therapist's job in second sessions in a way that is similar to first sessions. The therapist's job is to figure out what the client did that was useful or what happened in the client's life that the client could make use of. It's then the therapist's job to recognize the resources and competencies the client demonstrated by making these changes and to feed this information back to the client. If the client wants ideas about how to go on, the therapist can indicate what he or she thinks were useful things the client did and suggest that the client do more of them. The therapist can also suggest something the client hasn't tried yet but that fits with the way the client describes the miracle and the steps already taken.

When things are better, most solution-focused practitioners will also ask if things are "good enough" or "better enough." When the client answers "no," the therapist will generally ask what else needs to be better for it to be "better enough." When the client answers "yes," the therapist will frequently comment on this toward the end of the session or in the message after the break, saying something along the lines of "I am not sure you need to come back—what do you think?"

In her second session, Victoria has told Harry that she decided to change from "a devil without horns" to "an angel without a halo" and she has told him about how she broke up with the gang of girls that she was leading. She has also decided she wants to continue school and get into the science program at high school. It's 20 minutes into the session and Harry asks:

HARRY: I like your metaphor of being a devil without horns or an angel without the halo. You said you're at 6-7 on the miracle scale—so if 10 means that you're confident you can stay at 6-7 or at least be able to get up there again, and 0 means it's totally out of your control, where would you put yourself on that scale?

VICTORIA: I am both sure and unsure, because I could end up with the gang again, so I'd say 5-6.

HARRY: And what is it you know about yourself that tells you you're not at 0?

VICTORIA: Because I know I can do it and I have the will to do it.

HARRY: You know you can do it and you have the will?

VICTORIA: Yes.

HARRY: Is 6-7 minimally okay, is it okay the way it works now?

VICTORIA: Yes, it is not the best in the world but it isn't bad.

HARRY: Is it good enough for you to manage school the way you want?

VICTORIA: Yes.

What Else?

"What else?" is such an important question when using the miracle question and its scale, and the SFBT approach in general, that we want to emphasize it once again. When people in supervision show us tapes of their work and we ask them what they would have needed to do differently to get one step higher in how satisfied they are with what they have shown us, one of the most frequent answers is "more details."

Details aren't created automatically. You only get them if you listen actively and ask for more. Our solution-focused colleagues at the Brief Therapy Practice in London—Evan George, Harvey Ratner, Chris Iveson, and Yasmin Ajmal—say that it's when you've gotten to the fourth or fifth "what else" that you get the most useful answers (personal communication, 2000). So, let's imagine that you have been asking solution-focused scaling questions in reference to the miracle scale. Your client is at 3, and you've asked, "What else would be a sign that you have gotten to 4?" so many times that you feel that it's absolutely impossible to ask "What else?" one more time. That is exactly when you ask the question again: "What else would be a sign for you that you've gotten to 4?" We say this because it works.

We have offered many ideas throughout this chapter for asking the miracle question and its scale. We believe, however, that in the real-life environment of your own interviews, the most useful ideas will be yours, especially those that come to you as an immediate response to your client. Looking back upon the realities of your own work, what are some of your best ideas for using the miracle question? What else?

Chapter 5

The Friendly Stomach Discussion

The clients in this case are Robert and Robert's mother, Christine. The consulting therapist is Steve de Shazer, and Harry Korman is the colleague who referred the clients and comments at times throughout the session. The session begins with Steve asking the clients to tell him their names.

ROBERT: Robert.

STEVE: Robert.

CHRISTINE: Christine.

STEVE: Christine. Write your name. Then you *[gesturing toward Robert]* can write your name.

CHRISTINE: Yes.

STEVE: And then I can see if I can read it.

CHRISTINE: That could be difficult.

STEVE: *[Inaudible]* your name. Yeah. I know I can't read that. It's good practice for me.

CHRISTINE: *[Laughs.]* So.

ROBERT: And my name?

STEVE: Sure.

CHRISTINE: *[Laughs.]*

STEVE: I have to know which name you're using today, you now, so. Right. Okay. So, first, thank you for coming today. I hope that what we do will be—together will be useful. There's no guarantees about that. Huh. I can guarantee I will do my best. I assume you guys will too. And we see what happens. So, I know almost nothing. So, I imagine you were supposed to be going to school.

ROBERT: I am going to school.

STEVE: You are going?

ROBERT: Mmm-hmm.

STEVE: And what—what did the teacher say you were good at?

> Why do you begin by asking about what he does well instead of asking about the problem?
>
> Any solution has to fit into the client's everyday life. Otherwise, it will, of course, be rejected. So we need at least some details of this everyday life. Here the client is the expert and his competence can be put to use in taking steps he already knows about to build a solution.
>
> Of course the problem too is part of everyday life, but it is something the client wants to eliminate, so we want to construct things so that it becomes logical and reasonable for this competent person to do something different.

ROBERT: I don't know. I haven't been there for so long.

STEVE: Yeah.

ROBERT: It's . . . I'm new at school.

> Why is it better to find out about the problem later in the session?
>
> Once we've established that the client has skills, abilities, knowledge that helps him make it through each day, then these skills, abilities, etc. can reasonably be used to build a solution. This helps to establish a context in which it is reasonable to talk reasonably about problems. In fact, even people who are shy and uncomfortable about talking about their problems will bring them up when it is their right time. It's a therapist's office after all and it is the right place to talk about problems, so it will happen pretty spontaneously.

STEVE: Okay. Well, what do you think—the teacher's—you've been in school before. So, what . . . what do you . . . what did the teachers say you were good at in school?

ROBERT: Geography.

STEVE: Okay.

ROBERT: And math.

STEVE: Math, okay. And what do you think you're good at?

ROBERT: Math.

STEVE: Math. Okay. Good, good. And what is it you like about math?

ROBERT: I like the numbers.

STEVE: Numbers, yeah? Okay. So numbers somehow mean something for you?

ROBERT: Yeah.

STEVE: Yeah . . . Oh, okay . . . Good . . . Good. And Christine, how do you spend your days?

> Are you afraid of missing problems?
>
> I am more afraid of undermining what needs to happen in order for the solution to develop. And therapy to be over successfully.

CHRISTINE: I work. I work in a company. It's a bit, it's a bit of a way from here. And we have some *[Pauses, searching for the correct word in English, which is not her native language.]*

ROBERT: I can help you.

CHRISTINE: Yes. *[Laughs.]*

ROBERT: They—they . . . they do—you know the seeds you put in the ground?

STEVE: Mmm-hmm.

ROBERT: Create the seeds to put in the ground.

STEVE: Uh-huh.

CHRISTINE: Yes. Yes.

ROBERT: They produce that.

STEVE: Okay. So you grow seeds?

CHRISTINE: Yes. Yes, we do. Yes, we do.

STEVE: Mmm-hmm. Mmm-hmm . . . Okay. And is somehow this job good for you?

CHRISTINE: Yes, I have been working there for sixteen years. So, I think it's good.

STEVE: Mmm-hmm. And would your boss—your bosses say—think that you do a good job in your job?

CHRISTINE: Bosses never say that you do good job. They never say anything good.

STEVE: Yeah, I know that. But would they say—would they say if I were to ask them and they were to tell me?

CHRISTINE: Yes, I hope so.

STEVE: You hope so. How confident are you that they would?

CHRISTINE: Quite.

STEVE: Quite. Okay . . . good. Good. So—

STEVE: Yes. So far we're doing fine.

CHRISTINE: *[Laughs.]*

STEVE: So, I have my first question. You know these kinds of questions. So 10 stands for you've accomplished what you wanted to accomplish by working with Harry here.

At this point, not much has been said about the problem; do you worry about asking so soon about the solution? How do you know that you won't miss something important by not asking more about the problem?

As the session goes on, she will have to convince me that I need to know more about the problem in order for me to ask about it. . . . They will tell me about the problem or I will find out about it through scaling questions. The client naturally talks about the problem when necessary as part of describing the point that designates the problem and the solution on the scale.

CHRISTINE: Hmm.

STEVE: And you don't need to come and see him anymore. And 0 stands for how things were when you contacted him and said you know, can we come and see you. It's an arbitrary point. But, that's the point where 0 is. Where

We notice that you use 0 to symbolize the problem; why?

Zero implies that the problem is situated within a range (between . . . 1 and +1) and is therefore not immoveable. Putting the problem between two numbers like this suggests that it is something the client already knows and we are merely reminding him or her of it.

would you say things are between 0 and 10?

Zero as I see it is the beginning of therapy. Frequently things change a lot in the interval between the initial phone call and the first session. Since this is a consultation session, I think it is important to help the client let me and the therapist know that the therapy has helped things go in the right direction. Sometimes therapists do not know what a good job they have done, so this can be useful for them.

CHRISTINE: It had, it had been up and down.

ROBERT: Yes.

STEVE: Okay.

CHRISTINE: And . . .

STEVE: Today is . . . ?

Why do you ask about today? Why do you not focus more on the downs of the ups and downs?

Complaining about how bad things are is a social activity rather than a useful therapeutic activity designed to lead to a solution.

Although things have been up and down, the focus needs to be on today since we need to construct the next (small) step. We can always return to the ups and downs later in the session. But, when possible, I want to get as high a number as possible at this point to continue building the client's picture of competence.

CHRISTINE: Today, I think, because Robert has started onto new school . . .

STEVE: Mmm-hmm.

CHRISTINE: . . . and it's . . .

ROBERT: Three weeks.

CHRISTINE: Yes.

ROBERT: Yeah. Yeah.

CHRISTINE: And that's a good thing . . .

Is it possible that you are training the client to answer and think in a certain kind of way as a result of these questions?

Certainly. People talk differently at home than they do in the office, in a restaurant, etc. Each situation helps to determine what people talk about and how they talk about things.

STEVE: Okay. Mmm-hmm.

CHRISTINE: . . . for Robert. That's very good.

STEVE: Okay.

CHRISTINE: Because he has start 14 days and then problems come.

STEVE: Mmm-hmm. Yeah.

CHRISTINE: So, I hope we are going, it's going better.

STEVE: Yeah.

CHRISTINE: Yes. So, what should I say, 5–6?

STEVE: You're going to ask him . . . he has his own opinion.

CHRISTINE: Okay. *[Laughs.]*

STEVE: Right? And his might not agree with yours.

CHRISTINE: No.

STEVE: Okay. And you're saying?

CHRISTINE: Yes, 6.

STEVE: 6?

CHRISTINE: Maybe something a bit higher.

STEVE: 6 plus?

CHRISTINE: Yes. Yes.

STEVE: Okay, I can accept 6 plus. Okay.

ROBERT: 8.

STEVE: 8. Now, this raises a difficult question. If things were to continue at 6 plus and 8 for—I don't know—let's say six months. Would that be okay? Maybe not great, but okay?

CHRISTINE: Yes, okay. Yes.

STEVE: Mmm-hmm. Okay.

CHRISTINE: Because this has been going on for a long time, so . . .

STEVE: Good—good. And maybe you can tell me—I know you started because you've been in school for three weeks, but what else? What can you tell me about 6½ compared to 0?

CHRISTINE: Me or Robert?

STEVE: You.

CHRISTINE: Me. Okay.

STEVE: His is 8. We'll come back to that a little bit later.

CHRISTINE: *[Laughs.]* Okay. I think I see Robert is more—he has more—he's more . . . I don't know . . . satisfied.

STEVE: Mmm-hmm.

CHRISTINE: . . . with his life now. He feels better. He has not so much ache in his stomach.

STEVE: Mmm-hmm.

CHRISTINE: And he is, yes, he is smiling. He's, he is like almost a 17-year-old . . .

STEVE: Mmm-hmm.

CHRISTINE: . . . child. But when we started, he was not.

STEVE: Okay.

CHRISTINE: He had such big ache in his stomach. I don't know if that means that this school is making it different. I don't know.

STEVE: Mmm-hmm.

ROBERT: Well, it is.

CHRISTINE: But, I hope so. And I think, hope that it's going to be better time after time.

STEVE: Yeah. Yeah. Sure. Sure. He thinks it is better.

CHRISTINE: Yes. I do, I do also . . .

STEVE: Mmm-hmm.

CHRISTINE: . . . but I am a little bit *[inaudible]* . . .

STEVE: Cautious.

CHRISTINE: Cautious. Yes, I am. And . . .

STEVE: We should hope so.

This is interesting. Some therapists would have told her she didn't need to be so cautious or reassured her in some other way. When you agreed with her opinion instead of reassuring her, she suddenly became more positive and switched to talking about hope. Any ideas why this is so?

Of course if the therapist reassures her, she needs to defend herself and her idea. Things have been up and down and so she knows that things being up right now does not mean things will stay that way. Her experience runs counter to that, so caution is very reasonable. Once this is accepted she is free to express her hopes for the future.

CHRISTINE: Yes, but hope is . . . I think that's what you have to do. You have to hope.

STEVE: Yeah. Yeah. Um. So, there's something—you were saying before there's something different about this school. That he's there a long three weeks now?

CHRISTINE: Yes, that's, that's . . . that's long for Robert.

STEVE: Uh-huh.

CHRISTINE: This is the longest time for four years that this has been going on.

STEVE: And I'm going to ask him later.

We notice you do not allow her to speak for him. Why?

If one client speaks for another, the other might have answered differently, and I lose that piece of information which potentially might be key to the solution . . .

CHRISTINE: Yes.

STEVE: . . . How is he doing this?

CHRISTINE: Yes, how? I don't know. I don't know. I must say I don't know because he hasn't so much ache in his stomach and why he hasn't I don't know. He can get to school and he is satisfied with life.

They are both saying I don't know a lot, and yet the session continues? How do you do this? How do you work with clients who answer "I don't know" repeatedly?

Well, both therapists also say "I don't know" a lot during the session and I see "I don't know" as a serious, legitimate response to questions that clients find difficult. So, the best thing to do is to give the client space to think after this response before going on.

STEVE: Mmm-hmm. Okay. And so are you very . . . lots surprised or is it just a small surprise?

CHRISTINE: Yes, I am much surprised. Yes, yes, I am.

STEVE: Um. Good. Good. That's nice.

CHRISTINE: Yes.

STEVE: Yeah. So, you agree that being there for three weeks is somehow different for you?

ROBERT: Yes.

STEVE: Recently. Yeah. How . . . how are you doing it? How are you managing to stay in school for three whole weeks already?

ROBERT: I actually don't know. I just wake up. I don't have the aching stomach and I go.

This is the first time he talks about the absence of the pain, and this is a very different description than in the past where he talked about less pain. This leads to asking about what would be present instead.

STEVE: Mmm-hmm.

ROBERT: It's pretty simple.

STEVE: Yeah. Good. Good. Um. So, how come . . .

ROBERT: Have none.

"Suppose it were said: Gladness is a feeling, and sadness consists in not being glad. Is the absence of a feeling a feeling?" (RPP2, #159)

STEVE: When you wake up and you say you don't have this ache in your stomach? What do you have?

ROBERT: I have an ache, but I don't have it as much as before.

STEVE: Mmm-hmm.

ROBERT: It's less . . .

STEVE: Yeah. Yeah.

ROBERT: Than before.

STEVE: Okay. And how much less?

ROBERT: Pretty much less.

STEVE: Pretty much. Okay. We can do the scale with 10 being it's gone completely and 0 it's at its worse.

ROBERT: 7½.

STEVE: 7½. And that's a big improvement for you?

ROBERT: Yes.

STEVE: Okay.

ROBERT: It's a very big improvement.

STEVE: Okay. Good. Good. Do you have some ideas about what is happening or what is that much better?

ROBERT: What's causing it?

STEVE: To be better. Yeah.

ROBERT: I don't know. It just is.

STEVE: Isn't that a stupid question, what's causing it?

CHRISTINE: *[Laughs.]*

STEVE: . . .To be better do you think?

Wittgenstein suggests that an important question about feelings, such as feeling better, is: "In what sort of context does it occur?" (PI, p. 188)

CHRISTINE: Um, I don't know. But, yes, this three weeks, they haven't really studied the whole time. They had been together in small group of five, just five new, four new [students]. And the others were out doing some . . .

ROBERT: Practice.

CHRISTINE: Practice on *[inaudible]*.

ROBERT: But they are back now.

CHRISTINE: Yes.

STEVE: Uh-huh.

CHRISTINE: But it was the first day today. So maybe when . . .

ROBERT: That was great.

CHRISTINE: Yes, that's nice. That's nice. But, I hope that when homework and tests and so on . . . It's natural. When you get to school—

STEVE: Of course.

CHRISTINE: Yes. But when it starts, I hope Robert still doesn't feel he is—[that] he must do so very good at tests.

STEVE: Oh, I see. You think that he tries too hard on the tests?

CHRISTINE: Yes, I know he tries hard. And he wants to be one of the best.

STEVE: Sure.

CHRISTINE: Yes. That's always Robert's point.

STEVE: Good. Good.

CHRISTINE: But, sometimes when you haven't been in school for such a long time you have some loopholes.

ROBERT: Some holes.

CHRISTINE: Some holes.

STEVE: Sure.

CHRISTINE: And, I hope that it's going to be better. I hope it's going to work . . .

STEVE: Mmm-hmm.

CHRISTINE: . . . for him. I hope it's going to be all right for him.

STEVE: Okay. We'll come back to that in a minute.

CHRISTINE: Yes.

STEVE: Do you have ideas about how come his stomach is so much less painful? In your observations over the—

HARRY: That's, that's been sort of the mystery all along. That there have been . . . all along over the last year, it's been a year or something?

CHRISTINE: Yes, a year and a half maybe.

HARRY: Maybe more. I don't understand. I must have asked that question a hundred times. I don't have any idea what makes the difference.

STEVE: Mmm-hmm.

HARRY: Why he . . .

ROBERT: A thousand times.

CHRISTINE: *[Laughs.]*

HARRY: A thousand times. Okay. I must have spent at least 15 minutes every session asking that question.

STEVE: Mmm-hmm.

HARRY: And trying to figure it out with him.

STEVE: So there's something wrong about the question, maybe.

HARRY: Mmm-hmm. Maybe.

STEVE: Must be. Must be. So, let's change the question. Okay. What do you think you need to do or what needs to happen—both of those maybe—to make sure that it stays this way and doesn't get worse again?

ROBERT: I don't know. I cannot know. It's just either it's good or it's bad. I don't do something special about it. I don't know.

Is the client's confusion about knowing what he knows about himself an example of "the bewitchment of language?"

Perhaps. It is very difficult to talk about, to describe physical pain, particularly when it is so hidden away (in the stomach) that other people cannot see it. How can Mother talk about something she cannot see? There really are so few outward and visible signs of stomachache. So, she can only have some more indirect ways to clue her in. So, she might be able to only say: "He's in pain" or "He is not in pain," based on outward and visible signs, i.e., groans, etc. When he says, "I have a stomachache" he is sort of saying "ouch," which is just a remark—not a sign—which Mother has to accept at face value.

STEVE: Do you have some ideas?

CHRISTINE: I guess hope. Maybe it's hope.

STEVE: Mmm-hmm.

CHRISTINE: Yes, yes, I have. And I'm, I'm trying to take one day at a time.

STEVE: Mmm-hmm.

CHRISTINE: For a while every day you go to school. It's a miracle . . .

STEVE: Mmm-hmm.

CHRISTINE: I hope.

STEVE: Mmm-hmm. Mmm-hmm.

CHRISTINE: It shouldn't be [a miracle] because when you are 17, you should get to school.

STEVE: Yes, it's your job in life.

CHRISTINE: Yes. Okay. But . . .

HARRY: I think we can tell you some of the things we've tried.

STEVE: Oh, god . . . I don't want to do that now. No. I can imagine enough.

HARRY: He has a very irregular pattern.

STEVE: Mmm-hmm.

HARRY: You can imagine, yes.

STEVE: And you can correct me if I screw up too badly.

What do the clients know? The therapist doesn't know what they know and the clients don't know until they answer. In doing this, it is important not to lead, not to do a Socratic dialogue, but to really stay right there on the surface of what they are saying and find a way to ask the right question. If they cannot answer it, the therapist has either asked the wrong question or asked it in the wrong way. Oddly, therapy is a societal event in which the therapist is assumed to be the expert; however, in SFBT we try to find out what the client knows.

HARRY: *[Laughs.]*

STEVE: So, it's a mystery. Now another related kind of question, okay. How long would it have to stay at 7½–7 to convince you that the improvement was permanent? Or what other ways might—what other things might convince you that it's permanently better?

How did you decide to use the word *mystery* here? Afterwards Robert is convinced that it is permanently better, and the whole session seems to subsequently shift. How did you know to do this?

Everybody says "I don't know," so it is a mystery! Perhaps both therapists are being, have been, too logical and reasonable in their approaches, looking for ways to help the client take over some control of the pain. After all, if things get better by chance, then things can again get worse by chance.

ROBERT: I don't think I'll ever be convinced . . . believe it's permanently better.

STEVE: Mmm-hmm.

ROBERT: I will never become completely convinced, I think. Because it's been so bad . . .

STEVE: Mmm-hmm.

ROBERT: . . . with so much ache in my stomach that I don't think I will ever be convinced.

STEVE: Okay. What about more convinced rather than totally convinced?

ROBERT: A couple of years.

STEVE: A couple of years. Okay. Okay. Same question—that is the question, actually there's two there, yeah.

CHRISTINE: And I have been thinking.

STEVE: Good.

CHRISTINE: Yeah, um, and I think I would say the same as Robert says.

STEVE: Mmm-hmm.

CHRISTINE: That I don't dare to take too big steps.

STEVE: Right.

CHRISTINE: So, I just take small ones and hope that it's working out, that it's good.

STEVE: Mmm-hmm. Okay. So, how has he *[gesturing toward Robert]* behaved differently?

CHRISTINE: Now?

STEVE: When his stomach is feeling better compared to when he's feeling worse?

CHRISTINE: When he's feeling worse, he doesn't do anything. He just watches TV and maybe not more than that. He just sleeps and sleeps and sleeps.

STEVE: Mmm-hmm.

CHRISTINE: And, now he, yes, he is happy . . . happier. And he, yes, he can give you a hug and he, yes, he is . . . he's much more happy and then he goes to school and now yesterday you had some homework for today.

STEVE: Yes.

CHRISTINE: And he has done it. He has to. When he had some homework . . .

STEVE: Mmm-hmm.

CHRISTINE: . . . before and he was worse, he would say, "Yes, yes, I will [do it] soon . . ."

STEVE: Mmm-hmm.

CHRISTINE: "I can't. I'm so tired."

STEVE: Mmm-hmm.

CHRISTINE: But, now he does it by himself.

STEVE: That's a miracle. *[Turning toward Robert.]* Is that a miracle, too?

ROBERT: Mmm-hmm. *[Laughs.]*

CHRISTINE: I knew he wanted to do it.

STEVE: Mmm-hmm.

CHRISTINE: I have always known that he wanted to do it.

STEVE: Okay.

CHRISTINE: All . . . all the time.

STEVE: Mmm-hmm.

CHRISTINE: That is not the big . . .

ROBERT: Issue.

CHRISTINE: No, it isn't.

STEVE: Uh-huh.

CHRISTINE: Because I know that you really want to do good and want to do . . . But he just couldn't.

STEVE: Okay. Okay. Do you agree or . . . about that, the change in your behaviors at this point?

ROBERT: Yes.

STEVE: Compared to when the pain was worse?

ROBERT: Yes.

STEVE: Yes?

ROBERT: I slept most of the time.

STEVE: Mmm-hmm. What other changes in your behavior are noticeable?

ROBERT: Well, I am much more up to doing things. Like I would never hang out with my friends when I was [feeling] low.

STEVE: Mmm-hmm.

ROBERT: And now it's just . . . I hang out with my friends sometimes.

STEVE: Okay. And they notice something different about you?

ROBERT: I don't know.

STEVE: If they were here and I asked them. Do you think . . . what do you think?

CHRISTINE: I know what they can say.

STEVE: Okay.

CHRISTINE: I don't think they would say that they have noticed something . . .

STEVE: No. No.

CHRISTINE: . . . because Robert is very good to just keep his pain to himself.

STEVE: Mmm-hmm.

ROBERT: Hide.

CHRISTINE: What?

ROBERT: Hiding it.

CHRISTINE: Hide.

STEVE: Mmm-hmm.

CHRISTINE: To hide it, yes.

STEVE: I see. Okay.

CHRISTINE: So, other people who don't know Robert very . . .

ROBERT: Personally.

CHRISTINE: . . . personally as they don't—they don't see when he is hanging around with them that . . .

STEVE: Mmm-hmm.

CHRISTINE: . . . that he has this problem.

STEVE: Okay. Okay. I guess the big, main difference would be that they see you hanging around with them?

CHRISTINE: *[Inaudible.]*

STEVE: Mmm-hmm. Okay. And they accept you?

ROBERT: Yes.

STEVE: Mmm-hmm. Okay. Even though sometimes you're not there?

CHRISTINE: Yeah.

STEVE: So how come you're so lucky to have good friends like that?

This seems to be a very nice example of an indirect compliment that the client takes in by virtue of answering the question.

ROBERT: How come I'm so . . .

STEVE: Lucky.

ROBERT: Lucky.

STEVE: In having good friends like that?

ROBERT: I don't know. I actually don't know.

STEVE: Oh, well—okay. I get to ask all these wonderfully difficult questions and then they pay me for what you say?

CHRISTINE: *[Laughs.]*

STEVE: Okay. Well, let's see—you're saying things are at 8. Stomach is at 7½. Okay. So, how would you know on that scale—let's go back to that one—huh . . . that you have moved up to 9?

ROBERT: Well, the hurt just goes down. Ten it would be it doesn't hurt—ache at all.

STEVE: Mmm-hmm.

ROBERT: But at 9 it hurts very little—9 it just—it hurts.

STEVE: Okay.

ROBERT: A little less hurt—ache in my stomach would make it a 9.

STEVE: Okay. And so with less hurt, less pain in your stomach, what will you be doing at 8 and 9 that you're not doing now?

ROBERT: Probably nothing.

STEVE: So how would anybody know that you had gotten that much better?

ROBERT: As I said before, I'm very good at hiding . . .

Normally, in SFBT we look for external indicators, external reinforcers of the exception. We ask who would notice. But Robert's description of things being better is linked to a state that he literally feels inside his stomach. Oftentimes the problem with exceptions like this that are essentially feeling states, is that they are internal, not external. As Robert says here, his friends would not notice. Fortunately, Mom would notice. How do you decide what to do next in situations such as this where the client answers "I don't know" and both client and observer have described the solution as "feeling better"?

Usually feeling state questions do not lead to anything that is externally reinforceable, so I hesitated to focus on feeling better. In the early part of the session it came up as feeling "less" pain and then it came up as "not feeling pain," and the session began to shift. "It doesn't ache" is a very different statement than "It would ache less."

After questions following up on what would be happening when it doesn't ache, the client became more animated and intrigued. The description of the absence of pain made room for the therapist to ask what would be happening instead—the presence of something else instead of the pain—and thereby a description of the solution. Then it follows that the mother and brothers would notice this, and so you do have some external indicators, reinforcers.

STEVE: Mmm-hmm.

ROBERT: . . . my ache. So, they would probably not notice.

"Only surrounded by normal manifestations of life, is there such a thing as an expression of pain. Only surrounded by an even more far-reaching particular manifestation of life, such a thing as the expression of sorrow or affection. And so on" (Z, #534).

STEVE: What about Mother?

ROBERT: My mother would notice.

STEVE: Okay, what would she notice that would tell her he's gotten one step better?

ROBERT: I don't know. You have to ask her.

STEVE: I will. I want you now to guess.

CHRISTINE: *[Laughs.]*

STEVE: Because you know you and you know her.

ROBERT: Yes.

STEVE: So what would tell her that things are that much better? Because you don't want her to have false hopes. *[Pauses.]*

ROBERT: No.

STEVE: Okay.

ROBERT: I don't know what to say.

STEVE: Okay. What will tell you? You say less pain. But, I don't know how you know there would be less pain.

ROBERT: It doesn't ache.

STEVE: Yeah—what's there instead?

ROBERT: Happy feelings.

Interestingly, Wittgenstein thinks that "the world of the happy is quite another than that of the unhappy" (T, #6.43).

STEVE: Happy feelings. Okay. I shouldn't do this, but where do you have happy feelings? Can you tell me that?

ROBERT: Well, instead of an ache in my stomach, there would be happy feelings in my stomach.

Wittgenstein's questioner says "but 'joy' [an emotion] surely designates an inward thing." Wittgenstein replies: "No. 'Joy' [an emotion] designates nothing at all. Neither any inward nor any outward thing" (Z, #487). "Joy is manifested in facial expression, in behavior" (Z, #486).

STEVE: Okay. Okay. Because sometimes I think happy feelings are only in your face and smile. Okay, how about you? You were saying you're at 6 plus, huh?

CHRISTINE: Mmm-hmm. *[Laughs.]*

STEVE: And so how would you know you had gotten up to 7 plus?

More and more details of the solution, and information about the fact that Robert has a life come out in this section. Any advice about how to ask questions that elicit details such as this?

In some ways, details beget details. Here we are back to something he can know about unlike his stomachaches' ups and downs.

CHRISTINE. First of all that he has not so much ache, naturally.

STEVE: Mmm-hmm.

CHRISTINE: And then that he'd go to school every day, yes, and his work is nice and it's . . . it's good there.

ROBERT: It's going well.

CHRISTINE: Yes. And, yeah, and that Robert, as you say, happy feelings. I can see that happy feelings in his eyes and in his mouth and what you do.

STEVE: Mmm-hmm. Like?

CHRISTINE: Like?

STEVE: What?

CHRISTINE: Like what. Yes, like joking with his big brother and yes, having more [fun].

STEVE: Okay.

CHRISTINE: . . . and teasing with them.

STEVE: How much older is big brother?

ROBERT: Two and four years older.

STEVE: Oh, Two. Okay. And which one would he be joking with?

ROBERT: Both.

STEVE: Both.

CHRISTINE: Both, yes. *[Laughs.]*

STEVE: Okay. Which one has the better sense of humor?

CHRISTINE: Tony, the middle one.

STEVE: Okay. So he would know.

CHRISTINE: Yes, he would know.

STEVE: Oh, okay. I didn't know about him so I couldn't ask about that. So he would be the one who would know that he had gone up one step?

CHRISTINE: Yes.

STEVE: Because you would be teasing and joking with him more. Fighting with him, too? Or do you fight with the older one?

ROBERT: I fight with both of them.

STEVE: You fight with both of them?

CHRISTINE: *[Laughs.]*

STEVE: Equally?

ROBERT: Yeah, pretty much.

STEVE: Yeah. Yeah. Who wins?

ROBERT: Sometimes them, sometimes I.

STEVE: Yeah. Okay. So [turning to Christine] you must have a . . . with three of this age group, you must have your hands full: loud noise, loud music, and . . .

CHRISTINE: Yes, but it's nice. It's much . . . it's a much nicer time now.

STEVE: Mmm-hmm.

CHRISTINE: Because they have become easier than it was for three, four years before. Because, there were so many feelings in . . .

ROBERT: It was hell.

CHRISTINE: Yeah. *[Laughs.]*

STEVE: And so your brothers would agree?

CHRISTINE: Yes.

ROBERT: Yes.

STEVE: Okay. So they must be pleased by this, too?

CHRISTINE: Yeah. *[Laughs.]*

STEVE: Well, they might. They won't tell you *[addressing Robert]*. They might tell her, but they won't tell you?

ROBERT: No.

STEVE: Okay. Okay. So, if they were here, either one of them, I don't care. Um, what would they say about this? What might they tell us about what they think he needs to do to stay at the 7.5 on the pain? What does he need to do to maintain this level of happiness?

[Pause.]

STEVE: Yeah, well . . .

CHRISTINE: *[Laughs.]*

ROBERT: *[Laughs.]*

CHRISTINE: *[Laughs.]*

STEVE: Well, I'm just wondering. I don't know the answer to that either. But it would be nice if we could answer that. Because you know you have this improvement and . . .

ROBERT: It just is. It just is.

STEVE: Yeah . . . Yeah . . . Yeah. But . . .

ROBERT: There's nothing to do.

STEVE: Yeah . . . Yeah . . . Yeah . . . But, the problem with that is if you don't know how to maintain it, it could go bad again.

This seemed to be a time when you were very transparent with the client; you let him know why you were invested in finding out what he knew about how to maintain it. Any thoughts about when and how to do this with clients?

Actually, I was just thinking out loud here. Remember, this is a mystery we are dealing with and there still are missing and hidden clues. I do not think there are times when you "should" or "should not" do this sort of thing. Perhaps it is more useful when dealing with a mystery.

ROBERT: Then something has to happen before it can be bad again.

STEVE: Oh, yeah.

ROBERT: Yeah. Of course, there would be something that happens. I just maintain it right now.

STEVE: Yeah.

ROBERT: It is maintained. If something bad happens, of course, it will be bad, more bad. But, if something good happens, it will climb.

STEVE: Yeah.

ROBERT: But maintaining is just . . . maintaining is it. It just is.

STEVE: Yeah, but so, then you see, just maintain it and then it goes bad. The question is, if it goes bad, how do you bring it back up to 7½?

ROBERT: Hard work.

STEVE: Yeah. And that's why if we knew how you maintained 7½, then you would have the answer to that question. Oh, well. Are you lucky?

ROBERT: Sometimes.

STEVE: Sometimes. Is he a lucky guy?

CHRISTINE: Yes, when he hasn't the ache, I think he is.

STEVE: So do you think he's lucky enough to maintain this?

CHRISTINE: I hope so. Yeah, I hope. I must, I must hope that because . . .

STEVE: Well, hope . . . Yeah. Would you bet on it if you were a betting person?

CHRISTINE: No.

STEVE: No. Okay.

CHRISTINE: Definitely not. *[Laughs.]*

STEVE: That was what I was worried about. Yeah. *[Addressing Robert.]* Would you bet on it that you would maintain it?

ROBERT: Not a lot, but . . .

STEVE: Some?

ROBERT: Some.

STEVE: Not everything you have.

ROBERT: No, not everything. There's always that risk.

STEVE: Mmm-hmm. Okay. And if it were to get worse, would you know how to get it better again?

ROBERT: I don't think so.

CHRISTINE: No.

STEVE: That's what I was afraid of, yeah.

ROBERT: That's the next chapter.

STEVE: I'm sorry?

ROBERT: That's a later chapter. That's a later chapter.

STEVE: Yeah, I know.

ROBERT: Right now it's pretty good. I can go to school. I can do my studies. I can do my homework. I can be with my friends. It's pretty good right now. I don't know what to . . .

STEVE: Yeah. So, do you think—maybe, maybe here we're missing something. Do you think that just maybe doing your homework, going to school, smiling, teasing and joking with brothers . . . Did I miss doing the homework . . . I don't know if I missed that?

HARRY: Hanging out with friends.

STEVE: Hanging out with friends. If you continue to do those, your stomach will continue to stay better?

ROBERT: Yeah, I think so.

STEVE: Yeah. Okay. So maybe we're asking the question the wrong way. Okay. So how much time do you spend with your friends in the average week, let's say? In the last three weeks . . .

In fact, it seems this turned out to be a great question, but it made us think. . . . How do we know we are asking the question the wrong way? For example, if we don't get an answer that helps with the solution does that mean we are asking it the wrong way? Or could it mean we are asking the wrong question? Any hints for how to recognize when we are going in the wrong direction?

This is not so clear-cut. It is, of course, the response or answer that is important, not the questions. I guess the easiest way to say it is "If you do not like the answer, ask a different question." Certainly when things go in a circle, any different question might be useful. There is, of course, no need to say it like I do here. This is particular to how this session has gone.

ROBERT: In a week—well, nothing, but at the weekends . . .

STEVE: Uh-huh.

ROBERT: . . . it's pretty much.

STEVE: Uh-huh. What do you do with your friends when you're hanging around?

These questions seem to paint a more and more vivid picture of the exception times. You seem to do this in a very natural and comfortable way. Any advice about how to learn to do it?

I learned to do it through years of practice and years of watching other therapists work live or on videotape. Thus, my technique seems natural and comfortable because it has become second nature. Doing therapy is the only way to learn to do therapy, much like learning to drive a car can only be learned by driving a car.

ROBERT: Play computer.

STEVE: Okay.

ROBERT: Watching videos.

CHRISTINE: Watching videos.

STEVE: Watching videos.

ROBERT: Watching videos and playing . . . role-playing.

STEVE: Tell me what that is? What you're doing when you're doing that?

CHRISTINE: *[Laughs.]*

ROBERT: Oh, it's difficult. *[Laughs.]*

STEVE: Okay. I've got time. *[Laughs.]* Wait a minute. Wait a minute. Is this something you don't want to say in front of her *[indicating Christine]*?

ROBERT: No, it's okay.

STEVE: Oh, Okay. I forgot for a minute about her being here.

ROBERT: Yeah.

STEVE: Some things mothers shouldn't know.

ROBERT: Oh, that's okay.

STEVE: Oh, it's okay. Okay. Role-playing. Okay, but anyway, never mind. *[Inaudible.]* Tell me about it later. What else?

ROBERT: That's pretty much it.

STEVE: Do you and your friends spend time doing . . .

ROBERT: *[Inaudible.]*

STEVE: Doing homework together?

ROBERT: No.

STEVE: No, you don't do that?

ROBERT: We're not in the same . . .

STEVE: You're not in the same school. Okay. And, then how much time do you spend with your brothers?

CHRISTINE: The rest.

STEVE: The rest. Okay. And, what do you guys do?

ROBERT: Me and my brothers?

STEVE: Yeah.

ROBERT: Watching TV.

CHRISTINE: Playing computers.

ROBERT: Playing computers. *[Laughs.]*

STEVE: Okay. What's your favorite thing?

ROBERT: To me?

STEVE: To you, uh-huh.

ROBERT: Relaxing.

STEVE: Yeah.

ROBERT: *[Laughs.]*

CHRISTINE: *[Inaudible.]*

STEVE: And how would I know you were relaxing? What would you be doing that would tell me that?

ROBERT: I would be lying there on the sofa and just look at the television.

STEVE: Okay.

CHRISTINE: I have tried to say to him that he has to make something. So, he has . . . to move something and do some exercises or something because he has . . .

ROBERT: *[Laughs.]* That's rest.

CHRISTINE: Yeah. Yes, relaxing is just doing sometimes nothing.

ROBERT: *[Inaudible.]*

CHRISTINE: Yes.

STEVE: Okay. But, so far, he hasn't done this?

CHRISTINE: No.

STEVE: And if he were to do this, to start doing some exercise?

CHRISTINE: Yes, I . . .

STEVE: Would that tell you something?

CHRISTINE: Yes, it would. It would tell me that he's feeling better.

STEVE: Mmm-hmm.

ROBERT: But I don't want to exercise.

CHRISTINE: No, I know. But . . .

ROBERT: *[Laughs.]*

STEVE: Exercise is not usually a matter of wanting to. It's just about doing it.

CHRISTINE: Yes. But he had some little holiday for one week.

ROBERT: A week ago.

CHRISTINE: A week ago. And . . . it has been sunshine all the time nearly. And every day he has been out with his . . .

ROBERT: Friends.

CHRISTINE: Friends, and Tony.

ROBERT: My brother.

STEVE: Yeah.

ROBERT: Middle brother.

STEVE: Middle brother.

CHRISTINE: Middle brother, yes. And they have been playing football outside. And that was so nice to see . . .

ROBERT: And you were alone!

CHRISTINE: *[Inaudible.]*

STEVE: That's good for her, too.

CHRISTINE: Yeah, it's okay. But it doesn't matter really because . . .

STEVE: Oh, yes it does. *[Laughs.]*

CHRISTINE: I have seen that he has been out with his friends.

STEVE: Oh, okay.

CHRISTINE: And that was, it was nice.

ROBERT: That was because the sun was shining.

CHRISTINE: Yes. And it was in the holidays. So . . .

STEVE: Oh, okay. So, football playing comes and go with it, too?

ROBERT: Yeah, when it's . . .

STEVE: Yeah . . .

ROBERT: When it's sunny outside.

STEVE: Yeah . . . Yeah . . . Yeah. Sure. You're not going to do that in a snowstorm.

ROBERT: Yeah, you can.

STEVE: You can.

ROBERT: I've played in the snow before.

CHRISTINE: *[Laughs.]*

STEVE: Yeah. You must have been really feeling good then.

ROBERT: What?

STEVE: You must have been really feeling really good then.

ROBERT: Yeah, it was a couple of years ago.

STEVE: Oh. So, if it were to be snowing on Saturday—this coming Saturday—do you think you would go—could go out and play football?

ROBERT: Probably.

STEVE: Okay.

ROBERT: But I don't like snow.

STEVE: Yeah. I remember at your age we might go—go out and play basketball in the rain, snow.

ROBERT: That's nice.

STEVE: Yeah. Parents would . . . my mother, anyway, would get worried. "Oh, you're going to get sick." We never did.

ROBERT: *[Laughs.]*

STEVE: Yeah. Okay, so sometimes they go out and they do this football stuff. That's good to hear. It gives you some time to yourself.

CHRISTINE: Yes.

STEVE: Yeah. Which is good, too. And . . . and that encourages you on this that things are getting better when he does these sort of things?

CHRISTINE: Yes, it does.

STEVE: Mmm-hmm. Mmm-hmm. Okay. Good. Good. So is this the first—first time you've played football with . . .

ROBERT: No.

STEVE: No.

CHRISTINE: It's not so often.

ROBERT: In the summer I always did.

CHRISTINE: Yes.

STEVE: Mmm-hmm.

CHRISTINE: In summer, yes.

STEVE: Mmm-hmm. Okay. Okay. Good. So, you were saying before that at 6½ and 8, did that continue for two years or something that then you would be convinced that it was going to stay that way.

ROBERT: Right.

STEVE: That's a long time to wait.

CHRISTINE: Yes.

STEVE: Any ideas about what might convince you you don't have to wait two years? Either of you.

CHRISTINE: If I see that Robert goes to school every day and every day . . . okay, you can get sick sometimes.

STEVE: Sure.

CHRISTINE: But if you . . . you get on. You are home and then you get to school again and it's okay.

STEVE: Mmm-hmm.

CHRISTINE: Then I maybe have a little more hope . . .

STEVE: Mmm-hmm.

CHRISTINE: . . . to say that maybe it's going to be, it's going to stay that way.

STEVE: Okay. Okay. You know, he might be sick with some other kind of thing.

CHRISTINE: Yes.

STEVE: Then, so what. You know that happens to people.

CHRISTINE: Yes.

STEVE: Yeah.

CHRISTINE: And maybe that sort of thing, it's easier to take . . . then.

STEVE: Mmm-hmm.

CHRISTINE: . . . but in this way . . .

STEVE: Yeah. Yeah.

CHRISTINE: It isn't.

STEVE: Yeah, absolutely.

ROBERT: I'm doing fine right now.

CHRISTINE: Yes, and that's nice. That's very nice.

STEVE: Yeah. And it's very hard to tell because his stomach is sort of—it's sort of hidden away and you can't tell when he's got a pain in his stomach. It's hard to tell this. Yeah. Mmm-hmm. Okay. So, is it right that the more you see him playing football, the more he goes to school, the more the homework gets done without your having to nag him, and the more he's joking and *[inaudible]* and so on . . . As that happens, you become more and more confident that the improvement will continue.

This sounds like a summary, but in fact it is not because it is actually in the form of a question. However, the question lists the details of many exceptions, a series of small details you have been collecting throughout the session and are now putting together, and in so doing a picture is now painted of the solution and the client's life apart from the problem. Listing exceptions like this, rather than being a summary, is actually more like a confirmation, as if the therapist is asking, "Do I have this right?"

CHRISTINE: Yes.

STEVE: Okay. Okay. That's good. Clear enough.

Are these details you mentioned above external indicators of the solution?

Right. These things and other things more or less like them are the outward and visible signs of the solution.

CHRISTINE: And maybe I can believe in it, too.

STEVE: Mmm-hmm.

CHRISTINE: If it's going to work and it's going to be all right.

This was an amazing shift in comparison to how the session began. Her expectations have really changed. Any thoughts about how you got to this point?

I think it is a logical and reasonable conclusion, a natural and normal point to be reached as a result of this conversation.

STEVE: Mmm-hmm.

CHRISTINE: Because if no, he has to take one day at a time.

STEVE: No—yeah—yeah—yeah—absolutely. Yeah. Um. So is there anything I forgot to ask or you forgot to tell me about this improvement that comes into your head that might be useful or important for me to know?

CHRISTINE: I don't think so. *[Turning to Robert.]* Do you? No.

HARRY: Well, there's such a big difference between the desperation when we met last in January.

CHRISTINE: Yes. Yes.

STEVE: Do you sort of really . . .

CHRISTINE: Yes.

HARRY: And I'm thinking about what I said. I said I don't have the sense that I am of any help to you.

CHRISTINE: Um.

HARRY: And I sort of more or less told you, you guys, you've got to do something about this on your own and I offered this possibility to meet Steve. Did that make . . . I'm wondering if that's sort of . . . if you thought about that or if that hit you with something. And you've been pretty dependent on seeing me. At least you have, Christine.

CHRISTINE: Yes.

HARRY: I'm not sure about you *[addressing Robert]*, but your mother.

CHRISTINE: I'm taking . . . I have been taking everything to try to . . .

ROBERT: Every opportunity.

CHRISTINE: . . . help. Yes, to help Robert. My . . . sometimes it's, you have to listen to other people, other people who have been working with this thing that could help a lot.

HARRY: So when I said I can't help you, what did you do?

CHRISTINE: I went home and sat down and cried. *[Laughs.]*

HARRY: And what did you do after that?

CHRISTINE: And after that I said yes we have to try to . . . You have to hope that this meeting would give us something to believe in again, or something. Yes.

HARRY: Okay.

CHRISTINE: Do you know? Do you understand me what I mean?

HARRY: I'm not sure, but . . .

CHRISTINE: No.

HARRY: . . . Maybe Steve does.

STEVE: Yeah. One question came into my head that I want to ask. Is there a girl?

ROBERT: What?

STEVE: Is there a girlfriend in your life?

ROBERT: No.

STEVE: No. And if—when this happens, when you get a girlfriend in your life, what effect do you think that's going to have?

> How did you decide to mention the girlfriend?
>
> It seemed to me that this was the only big missing piece in his daily life and the mystery. Most of the time, young men of his age will at least have mentioned girls. So, I wondered.

ROBERT: Well, I certainly would be a lot more cheerful.

STEVE: Mmm-hmm. Would that . . . do you think that would have some effect on this getting better business?

ROBERT: Probably.

STEVE: Yeah. Oh. Okay. That was the only question to pop into my head while I was . . . *[Addressing Harry.]* Do you have any? All right. I think we should take a break and we'll be back in 10 minutes. Okay. Just relax.

CHRISTINE: Yes, we do.

STEVE: Okay. You need more practice in just relaxing. Just . . .

[Pause.]

STEVE: Well, I'm glad you both came today and I thought I saw some new talent that I hadn't heard about before today. *[Steve is referring to a picture Robert has been drawing on the office chalkboard during the break.]*

HARRY: I wrote down some of the stuff the team said about you.

CHRISTINE: Yes.

HARRY: And they are very impressed by how concerned you are and how caring you are and your perseverance. And you—at the same time being smart, taking one day at a time. But also, I mean you have been seeking help for four years.

CHRISTINE: Yes.

HARRY: And you never gave up. And it must—

CHRISTINE: I couldn't.

HARRY: Oh, sure, but it also must take some knowing about what is possible to sort of give you the power to continue to search knowing that you could.

CHRISTINE: Yes.

HARRY: Not believing that it's impossible. There's force in that. And at the same time being cautious at this point is a sign of wisdom. Okay. And someone pointed to the fact that you're very, very good at sharing your happiness about him being better and showing him that.

CHRISTINE: Yes, but I think that's . . . that's one of . . . [the things] that you have pointed out and you have tried . . . to tell me to do that sometimes when I just feel: "What shall I do, what can I do, how can I do?" And I think of what you are simply saying during these meetings we have had in 1½ years. And you have said, "Try to see the good things that was happening just now. And, my older sons, I think we are very close, and we are talking, and they are seeing when I am not feeling so well about everything and they try to kick [get] me there.

ROBERT: Kick you there.

CHRISTINE: *[Laughs.]*

HARRY: That's good. That's very good. That's very good.

STEVE: Yeah. Yeah.

CHRISTINE: *[Laughs.]*

STEVE: That's good. I'm glad to hear that. And, they wanted to say . . . wanted me to say about how impressed they have been also with your outstanding English.

ROBERT: Thank you.

STEVE: So . . . I think it's, you know . . . outstanding is a good word for it. Um. I was also impressed with your ability to observe things and your sense of humor.

ROBERT: It's pretty cheap, but it works.

STEVE: Yeah. Sure. It, you know . . . I think it would be a good idea to make sure that good things happen to you so that you can make . . . continue to make things better. I don't know quite how you do that, you know, but, because, you know . . . obviously from what you were saying, I agree with that. That, you know, when good things happen you feel better. Um. I was thinking that, you know, that when you

> But these "happy feelings" are new and the stomachache has been around a long time. The experiment might help the client remember that he feels "happy feelings" long enough for him to learn to automatically begin each morning with "happy feelings."
>
> Of course this experiment is just as vague as everything else in this session. Anything less vague stands a chance of being somehow "wrong" in the eyes of the client and thus the client will not find it useful should he decide to do it.

wake up in the morning and you have good feelings in your stomach, you should try to make friends with them.

ROBERT: Make friends with my good feelings.

STEVE: Mmm-hmm.

ROBERT: Okay. That sounds very weird.

STEVE: Yeah. Yeah. Yeah. But, they are somewhat new friends. And so, you know, you should get to know them as well as you can. Just spend five minutes or so every morning with them. Okay. Well, it's just an idea that I think might help—be useful. I don't know. So, again, I want to thank you both for coming today. I hope it turns out to be useful. You'll let me know at some point. That's all.

How did you decide on this message? It seems like you incorporated Robert's exact words. Is it important to use the client's exact words in situations like this?

By using the client's exact words I can show the client that I have indeed been listening. Even paraphrasing might suggest that the client had been in some way wrong and I do not want to do this.

HARRY: Hmm. Making friends with your stomach.

STEVE: Okay. So, take care of yourselves.

Does Mom have a role in maintaining the solution?

Mom is key to keeping the solution going.

How would you approach this if Mom wasn't here?

Perhaps, since Mom is so involved, if she had been absent, the focus might have been on his perception of her ability to perceive whether he was feeling better or not. I can imagine an experiment built around his trying to fool her into thinking things were better.

CHRISTINE: Same to you.

STEVE: Have fun. Okay. I guess I'm ready to . . .

HARRY: Do we set up an appointment some time later on?

CHRISTINE: Yes. I think we should since . . .

STEVE: Particularly to study how it maintains.

CHRISTINE: Yes.

HARRY: And how he's making friends. It's an interesting idea. I never thought of that.

CHRISTINE: Yeah.

HARRY: Thank you, Steve.

From a systemic perspective, some people might interpret his sickness as a response to his mother needing him to be at home. What do you think?

Theories like that are based on interpretation rather than observation and can lead therapists away from finding out information necessary to the solution. Furthermore, the mother has said that she hopes he will feel better. SFBT tends to take people at their word.

Is SFBT a therapy that only asks questions? Throughout this interview you ask question after question . . . Do directives, statements have a place in SFBT?

Directives, statements tend to pull the conversation away from what we are dealing with and contribute to developing strange ideas about people. Questions don't do this. Questions keep therapists right there . . . using questions prevents me from doing interpretations.

[End of tape]

Chapter 6

Don't Think, But Observe

Understandably, I (SdS) have often been asked about my interest in and frequent citation of Wittgenstein's work in both my writing and my training seminars in solution-focused therapy. Wittgenstein saw the philosophical problems that concerned him as involving traps or knots that are inherent within language. Of course, we must use language to battle the bewitchment of these traps and knots. Since SFBT and most other therapies take a conversational form—therapy, like philosophy, is done within language—therapists and clients are subject to falling into the same and similar traps, and to getting all tied up in the same kinds of knots. Obviously, language is the primary tool of clients and therapists for doing therapy, and language must be used to resolve muddles and to get us out of the traps and knots inherent in language.

Since I maintain that SFBT is a practice or activity that is without an underlying (grand) theory, it may seems at least strange if not contradictory to refer over and over to a philosopher's work. This mistakenly leads some readers and seminar participants to the idea that Wittgenstein's work might actually provide the theory deemed missing in SFBT. However, as they quickly discover if they are looking for a philosophical system or theory, reading Wittgenstein is at the very least disconcerting and confusing since he does not provide such a system or theory. Rather, his work is "non-systematic, rambling, digressive, discontinuous, interrupted thematically and marked by rapid transitions from one subject to another" (Stroll, 2002, p. 93). This means that the reader has to work hard to follow the crisscrossing of the various threads of the argument. Wittgenstein deliberately uses this approach in very subversive and strategic ways designed to make the reader *look again* and thus think in new and different ways.

It might not be overstating things to call Wittgenstein the greatest philosopher of the twentieth century. His work is certainly different from that of any other philosopher. Many people inside and outside the field of philosophy have given him the label of "genius," starting with Bertrand Russell. For instance, Stroll (2002), who calls him "the greatest modern philosopher," says that

> the later Wittgenstein stands at the end and outside of that [philosophical] tradition and can be thought of as turning it on its head. The tradition sees the ordinary person as confused and in need of philosophical therapy. Socrates is the paradigmatic philosopher on this view. He walked around Athens questioning his fellow citizens and quickly exposed the shallowness and inconsistencies of the thinking about fundamental issues. For Wittgenstein the emphasis is in the other direction. It is philosophers like Socrates and his successors who "tend to cast up a dust and then complain they cannot see" and who need help (p. 5).

Philosophy, from its very start over 2000 years ago, has focused on the perplexity and complexity of the individual, seeking insight into and understanding of the individual person and his or her inner processes and states. Philosophers sought the essence of the thing—"thought," "knowledge," "being," "object," "time," "I," "name," etc. Psychology, a relatively recent offshoot of philosophy, has continued this focus on the individual's mind, emotions, and behavior. Psychology, and its "cousin" psychiatry, has worked to understand what inside the troubled individual has gone wrong—provide a diagnosis—and how to fix it.

Wittgenstein looked at traditional philosophy's project in a quite different way:

> When philosophers use a word—"knowledge," "being," "object," "I," "proposition," "name"—and try to grasp the essence of the thing, one must always ask oneself: is the word ever actually used in this way in the language-game which is its original home?
>
> What we do is to bring words back from their metaphysical to their everyday use (PI, #116).

Wittgenstein, talking about classifications (such as diagnosis) in general, remarked that:

> The classifications made by philosophers and psychologists are like those that someone would give who tried to classify clouds by their shape (PR, #154).

For Wittgenstein, "everyday use" is the bedrock of his activity, his practice as a philosopher. For instance, he offers this approach to a traditional, philosophical puzzle:

> Compare knowing and saying:
how many feet high Mont Blanc is—
how the word "game" is used—
how a clarinet sounds.

> If you are surprised that one can know something and not be able to say it, you are perhaps thinking of a case like the first. Certainly not of one like the third (PI, #78).

Clearly, the various uses of the words "knowing" and "saying" are striking and obvious. The difficulty arises when we start to think that words carry their meaning around with them rather than seeing that meaning arises out of use. For example, knowing how a clarinet sounds and knowing the height of Mont Blanc are two very different uses of the word "knowing," and saying what you know in each case is a very different kind of activity. There is nothing mysterious here. We were all trained to use these words and we would not expect ourselves or anyone else to be able to say how a clarinet sounds. The mystery developed because philosophers traditionally wanted to find the essence of "knowing" and "saying" and therefore became confused when the words were removed from the contexts in which they normally are used.

In the course of his work, Wittgenstein seems to have had various targets in mind: "Nearly all the major problems of traditional philosophy—change, universals, abstract ideas, skepticism, meaning, reference, and mind—derive from the thought of Plato and Descartes" (Stroll, 2002, p. 105) as well as Kant's and Wittgenstein's own early work. As Williams (2002) puts it:

> For Descartes, both immediacy and intentionality are explained in terms of the special infallible knowledge that the thinker has of the contents of his own mind. This epistemological mark of the mental privileges the subjective over the public and/or social as the starting place for language, belief, and knowledge (p. 2).

This individualistic point of view, with the individual having a special, infallible knowledge of the contents of his or her own mind, is essential to traditional psychology and psychiatry. Furthermore,

> Wittgenstein is fundamentally opposed to the picture of mind according to which experience or knowledge is some kind of amalgam of given sensory data and active mental construction and operation. Wittgenstein repudiates the metaphysics of both a Cartesian and a Kantian variety. Grammar, rules, concepts are not the *a priori* metaphysical or epistemological conditions for the possibility of experience, judgment, and action. Grammatical propositions, rules, and concepts can be abstracted from our ongoing practices, from our language games, but they do not ground those games (Williams, 2002, pp. 3-4).

For most of the twentieth century and continuing in the twenty-first century, the concepts of traditional psychotherapy have been firmly grounded within the traditional philosophical framework. For instance, emotions have been seen as something inside the individual. Sometimes these emotions have been seen as triggering, perhaps even causing, an individual's behavior. (Certainly all of us at times talk about our emotions as providing a reason for doing what we did; this is a normal way of talking.) Thus, the psychotherapeutic emphasis has been on the individual's controlling or managing his or her emotions.

> Such mental-process accounts draw on certain misconceived propositions, such as sensations are private, acts of imagination are voluntary, people act on their intentions and beliefs, and so on. The propositions are misconceived, according to Wittgenstein, because they are taken as empirical claims describing interior states and causes of behavior. In fact, their status as grammatical propositions reveals them to be norms of our psychological language games. They are propositions like "The bishop in a game of chess moves diagonally." This proposition expresses a rule of the game, not an empirical claim about how bishop-shaped figurines move in the world. Sometimes they roll off the table (Williams, 2002, p. 10).

BUT, WHAT ABOUT THEORY?

> Theory is a system of concepts that aims to give a global explanation to an area of knowledge.
>
> —Wald Godzich (1986)

The term "theory" has many definitions and uses. In the seminars, workshops, and trainings sessions I have conducted in the past 20 years or so, therapists most often appear to at least implicitly use a definition similar to the one Godzich offered (above). Many therapists seem to want exactly this: a global explanation of SFBT. On the face of it, this is a quite reasonable request. After all, most if not all other approaches to therapy have a theory. Certainly this is true for the prototypical psychoanalysis. Freud's work offers a grand theory that can indeed be used to explain almost anything. Without such a theory of SFBT, therapists might well be afraid that they cannot stand their ground in discussions, arguments, and comparisons with more traditional therapists armed to the teeth as they are with highly regarded theories.

"But, what is the theory behind SFBT?" This question bounces around the seminar rooms, growing louder and louder over the years as interest in SFBT becomes more widespread. This question assumes that a theory must have come first, providing therapists who use SFBT with the certainty that formulas provide. Having a theory allows us to eliminate uncertainty. According to Bouveresse (1995), "[O]ne of the most consistent characteristics of Freud's enterprise is his remarkable conviction that it is enough to examine a single well-chosen case, or a very small number of cases, to know instantly what is necessarily fundamental and essential to all other cases" (p. 45). Thus, in Freud's dynamic theory, there is only one type of joke, one type of hysteria, one type of dream, etc.

According to Freud's theory, all dreams are wish fulfillments. "In the case of Freud [said Wittgenstein], a generalization is seized upon . . . dreams are not simply wish-fulfillment, they are fundamentally or in essence . . . wish-fulfillment" (Bouveresse, 1995, pp. 59-60).

In other words, if a patient's dream is analyzed, then at the end of the interpretation the therapist and patient will discover that the dream was a wish fulfillment. The next patient reports a dream and the therapist does an analysis but this develops into an interpretation that is not wish fulfillment. Does this mean that the theory was wrong and not all dreams are wish fulfillments? No, this means that, in some way or another, the analysis was wrong, because the therapist holds the belief that all dreams are wish fulfillments and, therefore, a mistake must have been made in the analysis. As Wittgenstein put it:

> Freud was influenced by the 19th century idea of dynamics—an idea which has influenced the whole treatment of psychology. He wanted to find some one explanation which would show what dreaming is. He wanted to find the essence of dreaming. And he would have rejected any suggestion that he might be partly right but not altogether so. If he was partly wrong, that would have meant for him that he was wrong altogether—that he had not really found the essence of dreaming (L & C, p. 48).

Something is wrong here. As Sherlock Holmes would say, facts can (do, should) change theory but theory does not—should not, must not—change facts.

Freud is generally regarded by therapists and the general public as a great theorist. In fact, he is often seen as one of the great minds of the twentieth century. However, he seems to build theory out of next to nothing. For example, witness Freud writing about his colleague Breuer: "The next question was whether one could generalize what he had discovered on the basis of a single case of illness. The state of things he had brought to light seemed to me so fundamental that I could not believe it would be absent in any case of hysteria, once it had been demonstrated in a single case" (Sulloway, 1979, p. 52). Essentially, Freud wanted to generalize to all cases of hysteria from one single case—and Freud talked about what he was doing as "scientific"!

> In Freud, the model of the dream-as-disguised-wish-fulfillment is not presented for what it is, namely a principle that determines the form of discussion of all the phenomena concerned, but as corresponding to the discovery of the real nature of dreaming: and it is applied to all dreams, not because it has been

> demonstrated by a scientific investigation of different kinds of dreams, but because it has been granted a privileged place in the discussion (Bouveresse, 1995, p. 47).

Thus, Freud's theory was not as scientific as he claimed it to be but rather it can be viewed as more of a mythology. Of course one could argue that there are other theorists who did not reason the way Freud did. However, one has only to look at Godzich's contemporary definition of "theory" to see how easy it would be to follow in Freud's footsteps. A "global explanation" easily becomes the essence of a field. But just by itself the term "global explanation" suggests the likelihood of generalizing from a small number of cases.

Wittgenstein has this to say about theory within his practice of philosoph y:

> . . . And we may not advance any kind of theory. There must not be anything hypothetical in our considerations. We must do away with all explanation, and description alone must take its place. And this description gets it light, that is to say its purpose, from the . . . problems. These are, of course, not empirical problems; they are solved, rather, by looking into the workings of our language, and that in such a way as to make us recognize those workings: in despite of an urge to misunderstand them. The problems are solved, not by giving new information, but by arranging what we have always known. Philosophy [and therapy] is a battle against the bewitchment of our intelligence by means of language (PI, #109).

He goes on to say that "the difficulty of renouncing all theory: [is that one] has to regard what appears so obviously incomplete, as something complete" (RPP1, #723).

Of course, eliminating anything hypothetical and all explanation means that therapists must work hard to simply stay on the surface of the conversation. All that is left is the conversation itself—listening and talking—and the description of the conversation looking into the workings of our language.

And again:

> Suppose people used always to point to objects in the following way: they describe a circle as it were round the object with their finger in the air; in that case a philosopher could be imagined who said: "All things are circular, for the table looks like this, the stove like this, the lamp like this," etc., drawing a circle around the thing each time.
>
> We now have a theory, a 'dynamic theory' of the proposition of language, but it does not present itself to us as a theory. For it is a characteristic thing about such a theory that it looks at a special clearly intuitive case and says: "That shows how things are in every case; this case is the exemplar of all cases."—"Of course! It has to be like that" we say, and are satisfied. We have

> arrived at a form of expression that strikes us as obvious. But it is as if we had not seen something lying beneath the surface.
>
> The tendency to generalize the case seems to have a strict justification in logic: here one seems completely justified in inferring: "If one proposition is a picture, then any proposition must be a picture, for they all must be of the same nature." For we are under the illusion that what is sublime, what is essential, about our investigation consists in its grasping one comprehensive essence (Z, #443-444).

Like many or even most theories, such a theory tells us how things must be or should be rather than telling us about or describing how things are. Describing and teaching SFBT practice demands that we focus on how things are so that the trainees can learn to do SFBT. It seems to me that only through learning to practice can therapists come to know SFBT.

Of course the tendency to generalize from one case to many or all can be overwhelming; it seems so normal and natural. Such a theory ignores the fact that things could easily be otherwise, and as Wittgenstein says, it is just a form of expression that seems obvious to us. Interestingly, the philosopher that Wittgenstein criticizes (above) who says "If one proposition is a picture . . . all must be of the same nature" is Wittgenstein himself in his early work.

* * *

Before we go any further, it might be wise to look at one of Wittgenstein's techniques.

> Compare → A newborn child has no teeth.
> A goose has no teeth.
> A rose has no teeth.
> (PI, pp. 221-222)

Pretty silly, isn't it? (Remember, Wittgenstein taught elementary school for a period of time.) My first impulse is to say that the third statement is obviously true. But, Wittgenstein was more sure about the second! Obviously the goose has no teeth in its jaw, but where—he asks—would you look for a rose's teeth? Now, do not be quick to reject the third assertion as nonsense. In exercises of this sort, he would suggest that we consider its opposite: A rose has teeth. In what context would this make sense? Well, we could imagine telling a story like this: A cow chews her food and subsequently, her manure is used to fertilize the rose, thus the rose's teeth are in the cow! This is not totally absurd because one can have no idea about where to look for teeth in a rose (PI, pp. 221-222). This example, perhaps a joke, points out the need to look at the context in order to understand a sentence. Without this context we cannot make sense out of the combination of words referring to teeth and a rose. This comparison also points out something we come across again and again in muddles of all sorts. Each of the three sentences shares the same form, the same grammar: X has no teeth. This automatically leads us to want to treat all three subjects in the same way: Babies, geese, and roses are all treated—at least for the moment—as creatures capable of having or not having teeth. We use the same logic in trying to verify each of the sentences. With some frequency this sort of normal, everyday operation leads us unexpectedly into knots and muddles.

Wittgenstein offers example after example of untying knots. He says:

> Language sets everyone the same traps; it is an immense network of easily accessible wrong turnings. And so we watch one man after another walking down the same paths and we know in advance where he will branch off, where he will walk straight on without noticing the side turning, etc. What I have to do then is erect signposts at all the junctions where there are wrong turnings so as to help people past the danger points (CV, p. 18e).

* * *

Wittgenstein applied what Fogelin (1996, p. 57) called his "three most fundamental ideas: the primacy of action over thought, the limits of explanation, and the identification of meaning with use" to a wide variety of topics ranging from pain to arithmetic to music and logic. The Viennese of his period certainly were more musically educated than most of us. (He reported to his sister that while in Berlin—studying engineering—he went to see Die Meistersinger 30 times!) He says "understanding a sentence is much more akin to understanding a theme in music than one may think. What I mean is that understanding a sentence lies nearer than one thinks to what is ordinarily called understanding a musical theme" (PI, #527). How many of us would present understanding a musical theme as something we would expect of our readers? How many contemporary readers would find the analogy more puzzling than useful? To put it another way: A note, a chord, a phrase, or even a theme from Mahler's 6th (for instance), no matter how individually striking, is only meaningful within the context of the whole of Mahler's 6th. The whole is not only both different from and greater than the parts; it defines the parts. Outside of its home it loses its meaning. Similarly, when words and sentences are removed from their home—a language-game or the everyday activity of speaking a language—their meaning can easily get lost.

Facts

Early in the Tractatus (T) Wittgenstein sets the stage for much of his work with the concept of "facts," stating that the world is the totality of facts, not of things, and it breaks down into independent facts that divide the world up. A "fact" is a thing within its surroundings or context. According to Wittgenstein's early work, the pictures of facts are mirrored in language to give us meaning, so that we can say truly a hippopotamus is not in the room. Of course, a fact can always be otherwise. We can imagine a hippo in a room.

Family Resemblance Concepts

Philosophers, psychologists, and therapists constantly see the method of science as a model and are thus tempted ("tempted" is not really a strong enough word!) to ask questions and seek answers in the way science does. Perhaps because of the scientific model, we almost feel compelled to study language as an abstract system rather than as an activity. However, as Wittgenstein puts it, this "leads the philosopher [and, I add, the therapist] into complete darkness" (BBB, p. 18). This preoccupation with and devotion to the method of science leads philosophers and therapists to desire and even demand that "the explanation of natural phenomena [be reduced] to the smallest number of primitive natural laws" (BBB, p. 18) via unified concepts and simple causal connections. As Wittgenstein put it:

> The insidious thing about the causal point of view is that it leads us to say: "Of course, it had to happen like that." Whereas we ought to think: it may have happened like that—and also in many other ways (CV, p. 37e).

However, most of the concepts therapists and clients actually use in our day-to-day work are not of the scientific, artificial, unified type; rather, they come from our everyday life. The concepts we actually use involve "a complicated network of similarities overlapping and crisscrossing; sometimes overall similarities, sometimes similarities of detail" (PI, #66) that Wittgenstein called "family resemblance concepts."

The concept of "game" can be used as a prototype. Various activities we call "games" such as basketball, tennis, golf, and solitaire "have no one thing in common which makes us use the same word for all—but . . . they are related to one another in many different ways" (PI, #65). As a further example, take the word "good." What is common between a good joke, a good tennis player, a good man, feeling good, goodwill, good breeding, good-looking, and a good-for-nothing? The word "good" does not seem to refer to a specific entity or even a common property. However, because of its uniform appearance, we automatically assume it refers to an entity or a common property about which we can generalize. We take it out of its context, out of its natural place in talking and view "meaning as a halo that the word carries round with it and retains in any sort of application" (CV, p. 44e). Goody-goody, good grief (Charlie Brown), good weather, good taste, tastes good, good day (usually said "g'day"), a good buy, good-bye, etc. By looking at example after example, we eventually come to realize that there is some sort of vague family resemblance among the various uses of the term. There are certain features in common but there are no strict boundaries; a non–family member might have "the same nose." In other words, "the formation of a concept has, for example, the character of limitlessness, where experience provides no sharp boundary lines. (Approximation without a limit.)" (RPP2, #636).

Language-Games

What Wittgenstein calls "language-games" can be simply described as slices of everyday life, the home base of words and concepts. He describes language-games "in three ways: As a methodological tool in examining philosophical theories, as akin to the way in which children learn [training], and as an explanatory device describing language use in relation to other forms of acting" (Williams, 2002, p. 220). These are the everyday practices and activities in which words are used that provide words with their meanings. Wittgenstein lists several as examples within his definition of the term:

> The term "language-game" is meant to bring into prominence the fact that the speaking of a language is part of an activity, or of a form of life.
>
> Review the multiplicity of language-games in the following examples, and in others:
>
> Giving orders, and obeying them—
> Describing the appearance of an object, or giving its measurements—
> Constructing an object from a description (a drawing)—
> Reporting an event—
> Speculating about an event—
> Forming and testing a hypothesis—
> Presenting the results of an experiment in tables and diagrams—
> Making up a story; and reading it—
> Play-acting—
> Singing catches—
> Guessing riddles—
> Making a joke; telling it—
> Solving a problem in practical arithmetic—
> Translating from one language to another—
> Asking, thanking, cursing, greeting, praying (PI, #23).

As Wittgenstein points out over and over, the everyday use of words is a social, interactional, activity.*

---

*"Commanding, questioning, recounting, chatting, are as much a part of our natural history as walking, eating, drinking, playing" (PI, #25).

Chapter 7

My Real Self

I (IKB) was busy getting ready to begin the lecture to teachers and invited guests from the school district in the Garza Independence High School auditorium one winter morning. A good-looking African-American student walked up to me and offered me assistance. He asked if there was anything he could do to help me. Surprised and delighted at this offer, I began chatting a bit and this young man started talking to me in Japanese. I was surprised and caught off guard, but we exchanged a few words about his dream to visit Japan some day.

Then out of nowhere, this young man, named Carl, blurted out that he tried to kill himself the previous night. Somehow the words were said in a wrong context; it took me a while to comprehend what he was saying. Then, to convince me about what he said, he stretched his neck and showed me a superficial scar, explaining that this was where he tried to cut himself. I could see the people drifting into the auditorium, so I proposed to him that we talk together after the lecture was over. He readily agreed and then went and found a seat for the morning's lecture.

Fortunately, a camera technician was making a documentary about the Garza School and he agreed to change the program slightly and videotape my interview with Carl. Even more fortunately, Carl lived only few blocks from the school and his mother was available to give us the consent to videotape my conversation with Carl. I did not have an office space at the school because I was just visiting for the day, so the interview took place in a corner of the school library.

INSOO: Uh, Carl, what is your best subject in school?

CARL: My best subject so far anyway has to be math, or Algebra II.

INSOO: Math and algebra?

CARL: Or just Algebra II, period.

INSOO: Algebra II?

CARL: Yeah.

INSOO: Oh, what's Algebra II? It's been a long time since I took algebra.

CARL: Well, it's like, kind of like a process. When you're in junior high, you take pre-algebra. It's like written math, kind of like, you use factoring, solving, grouping. It's basically like process of elimination and all that.

INSOO: Oh.

CARL: And then you move up. Like when you get to high school.

INSOO: Yeah.

CARL: You'll take Algebra I, the actual algebra. Then you take geometry, which I don't like. *[Laughs.]* And then you take Algebra II.

INSOO: Oh, so that's what you're taking now?

CARL: Yeah, and I like it.

INSOO: And that's what you're best at?

CARL: Yeah. I'm making all A's in it.

INSOO: You're making all A's in it?

CARL: Yeah.

INSOO: So you must be a very smart young man.

CARL: *[Laughs.]* Well, no. No, I'm all right.

INSOO: You're all right?

CARL: Average.

INSOO: Oh, I see. Okay. All right. Good. So math and Algebra II. So you're good in math also.

CARL: Somewhat, but I think if I were to major in something, it would probably be algebra or Algebra II or something like that.

INSOO: Okay. I wanted to follow up on what we got started just a little bit. We didn't have much time to talk.

CARL: Right.

INSOO: We had five minutes to talk this morning. So I want to follow up on that. You were saying that you wanted to . . . you wanted to kill yourself yesterday?

CARL: Yes.

INSOO: Yeah.

CARL: Um, pretty weird story actually 'cause, um, yesterday was just an ordinary day for me. I mean, 10:45 hit; I'd just finished watching *American Idol* earlier, and then I watched the president's speech and all that. And then I tried to go to sleep, but my brother, he keeps bothering me. And my brother, he just got out of jail. He's nineteen.

INSOO: He's nineteen, and he just got out of jail. Okay.

CARL: . . . and so he kept on bothering me to put on his favorite CD or something. I was like, no, I need to go to sleep; I need to go to school in the morning.

INSOO: Yeah.

CARL: So. Well, it didn't work out like that. So I got up; I knocked on my mom's door, and I told her, I said, "Can you please put the CD player up in his room so he can stop bothering me?" So he started using profanity at me or whatever. And then I used it back, a lot. And then I tried to calm myself down by going outside and trying to walk. But when I was walking, I saw a bus sort of come by, so I started running to the bus. I got on the bus, and I told the bus driver, I said, "I don't have any money to pay for the bus. If you can just let me go, I'm in some trouble right now." He says, "Sure, we can do that." So he gave it to me, the transfer. And I caught the bus to my aunt's house, Aunt Jasper. And while I was walking over there, I feel like this dark cloud over my head, and it was pitiful. Everything from love, hate, anger, frustration just collided. And when I went in there, I went in the kitchen. I rinsed off the knife, a big knife. And, luckily it wasn't sharp enough 'cause I held my head back while my aunt was right there. She was, you know, intoxicated, but she wasn't paying me any mind or anything. And I leaned my head back.

> Some therapists would immediately follow up on the dark cloud, but you did not; how come?
>
> I want to first join around competence and establish some examples of his competence and history of ability to make good decisions for himself before engaging around the problem. I can always return to the "dark cloud" by asking about it later if necessary, but typically I will learn the information I need spontaneously in the course of an SFBT interview.

"Conversation flows on, the application and interpretation of words, and only in its course do words have their meaning" (Z, #135).

INSOO: So she didn't see you doing this? Or she saw you, and it just didn't register?

CARL: It didn't register to her.

INSOO: It didn't register to her.

CARL: Until I held back my head and said my last prayers or whatever. And then I just started cutting; and you can see right here.

> On the videotape, Carl's tears are visible. Did it cross your mind to ask him directly about them here or later?
>
> His tears seemed completely understandable to me under the circumstances. Therefore, there is nothing to ask about.

INSOO: Yes. Yeah. Yes, I can see that, yes.

CARL: . . . and I'm just lucky to be alive today. You know, to speak about this because had I not known there was a sharper knife next to it, but I went for

> "I'm lucky to be alive today" does not reflect a suicidal mind-set. Can you talk about how you knew to go in this direction and why you did not follow traditional suicide interview protocol regarding lethality assessment, or begin talking about suicide contract?

that knife 'cause it was the biggest.

The information needed for suicide assessment comes out naturally and gradually in the interview. As it turns out, Carl had last night violated an existing suicide contract, so it apparently did not help.

INSOO: Yeah.

CARL: So, I thought I would have done more damage or something.

INSOO: Right.

CARL: So I just, I don't know; I thank God every day, you know.

INSOO: So, what helped? What helped so it didn't go through?

CARL: It's, I mean, I don't know. I mean, when I was—the knife wasn't—it wasn't that sharp, it was like a butter knife or something.

INSOO: Yeah.

CARL: It was just, you know, and so I made it to where it could cut harder, so I used force actually.

INSOO: Yeah.

CARL: So.

INSOO: And you're saying this is not the first time. It has happened other times as well.

CARL: It's happened other times, but this is the worst.

This is an example of getting information to assess Carl's level of safety without doing a formal suicide assessment.

INSOO: This is the worst it's been.

CARL: Yeah. Other times it's been like, burn myself with an iron or something, like right here.

INSOO: Yeah. Wow.

CARL: . . . or something like that.

INSOO: Yeah.

CARL: I mean, I would get all kind of thoughts in my head . . .

INSOO: Yeah.

CARL: . . . that I, you know, I just pray to God that I wouldn't think of them anymore. They just, you know, they just come around whenever, you know, I'm feeling depressed or something, you know, suicidal, you know.

INSOO: Okay. So, how did you manage to get to school today?

CARL: Well, that's a long story, too.

INSOO: What a night . . . I mean it was a terrible night you had.

CARL: Way terrible night.

INSOO: How did you show up in school on time?

CARL: Well, it's kind of great actually, 'cause while this whole conflict happened, I was at my aunt's house . . .

INSOO: Yeah.

CARL: . . . and they wanted me to stay the night. They said, you need to rest or whatever.

INSOO: Yes.

CARL: I said no, I want to go back home so I can get up and go to school in the morning.

INSOO: Oh my goodness.

CARL: 'Cause I haven't missed a day in school yet. At least —well, two days, but those were counted you know. as, you know, I was here.

INSOO: Yeah.

CARL: As I would go to the doctor or something.

INSOO: Yeah.

CARL: But I've been on a perfect attendance, you know, roll twice already.

INSOO: But some terrible night like last night, you still showed up in school.

CARL: Yeah.

INSOO: And you were helpful to me; you're trying to be helpful to me today . . . this morning. And you even participated in the group with a large group of people.

CARL: Large.

INSOO: A very large group of people. You are very outgoing, very bright, very articulate. I was just absolutely astounded when I saw . . . what I heard this morning and now, 'cause I didn't get a chance to talk to you because we were so busy. And you were just able to sort of set that aside.

CARL: Right.

INSOO: And you were going on and participated with what's going on.

Wittgenstein suggests how putting on a "happy face" might be useful when his questioner asks: "How long have you been happy?" A peculiar question. But it might make sense. The answer might be: "Whenever I think about it" (LWPP, p. 2e).

CARL: Yeah, but, I put on my happy face. Yeah, that's what I call it.

INSOO: That's what you call it?

Some therapists might have automatically assumed that the happy face was not real or asked questions based on an assumption or interpretation that something else was "behind" it; however, you did not question this, but allowed him to continue talking.

CARL: Yeah. I mean, it's not being fake or anything, but there are some people in this world you can't see through them.

INSOO: Yeah.

CARL: But sometimes you can know what they're going through, so what I try to do, I will tell people what happened, but still, I'll try to keep a straight face about it.

INSOO: Okay.

CARL: So, you know, whenever, you know, that thing we had today, I was listening to you, I was listening to what you had to say.

INSOO: That's what I thought. Yes, you were.

CARL: I was, you know, cooperating.

INSOO: Yes, you were.

CARL: So the whole thing about me cutting myself last night, that was, you know, that just blew me over when I was listening to you with the whole, you know, conversation, about how, you know, the school curriculum is going. How AISD [Austin Independent School District] is, you know, well, Texas in general, is you know, just—I don't know if I should say this—but they kind of crazy. I mean, I don't know. Well, yeah.

INSOO: So, in spite of that, when I first met you this morning, you approached me.

CARL: Right.

INSOO: And you were just so sociable, so friendly. Because I didn't know anything about this, about what happened to you last night. You're very outgoing, so personable and so friendly, and you asked me whether you could help me, is there anything I can do for you?

> In this case you preface a question with a compliment, so that it looks like a question, but in fact is a very nonintrusive form of compliment as well, because the client naturally acknowledges the compliment by responding to the question, but doesn't have to acknowledge it directly or thank you for it.

CARL: Yeah.

INSOO: I mean, you came to me with such an offer, trying to be helpful. I was just for a while, when you told me that, I thought, "No, he's just joking. He's pulling my leg." That's what I thought. But I wanted to make sure I had a chance to talk to you today, because of that. So apparently, life is not that . . . I mean, life at the family . . .

CARL: Is not easy at all.

> Without directly calling attention to the fact that Carl has already had tears in his eyes at times during this interview, you acknowledge his pain. You decide to express empathy by saying "Life is not easy for you," rather than by asking him what his tears mean.

INSOO: Is not easy for you.

CARL: No. I'm surprised I made it here today at school—well, not surprised, but then again, I'm actually glad to be here right now because instead of my home being you know, just a couple of blocks away from here.

INSOO: Right.

CARL: This school is my home because I come here to learn, I come to you know, to succeed. You know, to graduate, 'cause you know, I want to get that out of the way. Well, yeah, get that done with because some of my family, they, you know, most of them didn't graduate from high school. And one went to college, but she got pregnant at college so she dropped out. So, I really want to be like the first to go all the way at least.

INSOO: All the way to college?

CARL: All the way.

INSOO: And finish?

CARL: Yeah.

INSOO: I see. so, is your family supporting that idea?

CARL: My mom, she's been on me 100 percent.

How is it that you chose to focus on Carl rather than immediately bringing his mom in?

Since this was potentially a crisis situation, I did not have time to wait for the next appointment with his mom. Also, we will utilize his relationships with Mom through relational questions as the interview progresses.

INSOO: She is . . .

CARL: Yeah. And she was telling me everything like, the cap and gown situation that's coming up in February. And she was like, "Well, what are you going to get?" "I don't know, just the cap and gown and some invitations." She goes, "No, I'm going to get you a ring, I'm going to get you this and that." I go, "Well, Mom, bills are tight now. I mean, do you think you could handle it?" You know, so, but she was like, "No, you're my son, I'm going to do this for you."

Do you worry that by not addressing Mom's incompetence, you are encouraging him to depend on a parent who is not dependable?

Carl is 17 and obviously knows he has to help himself in difficult situations rather than depending on his mom. For example, he did not depend on her last night by going outside his house for help.

INSOO: My goodness.

CARL: I was like, okay, Mom, I mean, yeah.

INSOO: So she is behind you. She is very supportive of you.

CARL: Yeah.

INSOO: Okay.

CARL: And even when she found out today what happened, she was still strong about it. She knew, you know, that I was on the edge, you know.

INSOO: So. I'm amazed by this. You could have gotten into a big fight with your brother . . .

CARL: Oh yeah.

INSOO: Last night.

CARL: Oh yeah.

INSOO: So what made you decide you were just going to get out of there, walk away from that? And just get out the door, instead of staying there, in a fight? And you know, you probably would have gotten into big trouble, right?

CARL: Oh, everything. I just react to what's in my body. I just say, like if I get into it with somebody, I need to go somewhere to cool off, for a while. So . . . so, instead of just cooling off for a minute or two and then coming back and try to solve something, I usually try to stay off for like an hour or two, you know.

INSOO: Yeah.

CARL: Just to get, you know, just get it all out, you know: my frustration, you know, crying, you know, all that emotion.

INSOO: So, is this something you learned? Or someone taught you? Because many kids, many young people don't know how to walk away; they just hang in there, and they get into trouble, a lot of trouble, and become violent and you know, things like that. So, how did you know that it was time to walk away?

CARL: I just knew. I mean, ever since I was younger I always knew to walk away.

INSOO: Is that right? You knew, since you were young?

CARL: Yeah, 'cause me and my brother, we had you know, we were at it for a while, a whole while. I mean, by him being in and out of jail, or a treatment center. He would always come back the same person, and I would always hate that because you know, I was expecting a change in him.

INSOO: Right.

CARL: 'Cause I always remain the same, except now I'm more firmer, and I stand my ground now.

INSOO: Yeah.

CARL: 'Cause I used to let people run over me. You know, tell me, well, you got to do this and that, you know.

INSOO: Yeah.

CARL: So now, I'm sort of in control, but then again, you know, everybody needs to be in control of their life at a point.

INSOO: Absolutely, everybody, of course, of course. You have to be in control. So you were being very assertive last night with your brother?

CARL: Right. Very assertive.

INSOO: Very assertive.

CARL: I mean, people, if they would like, my friends from Garza or the facilitators were there, they'd be like, "Is that Carl, or . . . ?" *[Laughs.]*

INSOO: Is that right?

CARL: "Is that somebody else?" Yeah, because I don't usually act like that whenever—yeah. If I get into it with somebody then some stuff is going to come out, all my anger, everything comes out. But I'm a pretty stable person. I mean, I reason with people, but a person like my brother, you know, my blood, is kind of hard to, you know . . .

INSOO: Yeah.

CARL: . . . reason out with him.

INSOO: Yeah, it's hard to do that.

CARL: Yeah, because he's, you know, mental, a little; he was born premature.

INSOO: Yeah.

CARL: And my sister, she has a mental problem, too, but she's not willing to admit it. But I told them, I said, forget them, because they tell me, "Oh, why did you go Shoal Creek Hospital?" or something like that. I said, "Well, that's me, I'm getting help for me. I don't care about you. Well, I care about you in a loving way, but as in, you need to respect that I'm trying to get help."

INSOO: Mmm-hmm. Mmm-hmm. Wow, so you've been thinking about this for a long time?

CARL: Oh yeah.

INSOO: A long time. And last night it sounds like, your being assertive was helpful for you.

CARL: Right.

INSOO: Right. But somehow you weren't . . . quite didn't know what to do with it after that . . . after being assertive.

CARL: Right.

INSOO: So, you went to your aunt's house. And that wasn't very helpful.

CARL: No, that wasn't very helpful. I mean, when I was on that bus, I was just thinking, the first thing I'm going to do is go off in there and do something crazy, like try to kill myself. But then, on the other hand, I kept on thinking of all the people I would hurt if I do that, you know. I wouldn't live; I wouldn't see my graduation. I wouldn't, you know, see my family grow. So, those things just combined and just . . .

INSOO: Right. So you decided that you were going to live. It's better for you to live than die?

CARL: Yeah. I went through it, but I came out of it all right.

INSOO: Yes, you have. Yes, you have. I'm very glad about that. Right. So, there is a change for you, what you did last night? Compared to what you used to do in the past when you were faced with such a difficult decision?

CARL: It's a yes and a no.

INSOO: Okay.

CARL: What happened last night made me realize that I need to be more aware of myself because sometimes I'll get too carried away, or I'll try to calm myself down. The majority of the time that works, but something so deep and dark that hovers over me, I have no other choice but to you know, just rid myself, you know, which is wrong. I know it's wrong.

INSOO: Yeah.

CARL: And I don't ever want this to happen again.

INSOO: Okay.

This is a really nice example of how Carl's current state is much different than how he felt last night. He clearly does not want to get hurt.

CARL: But sometimes those thoughts come into your head, saying, you know, "You're not good."

INSOO: So, is that what happened last night? Something told you that you're not good?

CARL: Something told me, yeah.

INSOO: Is that when you tried to hurt yourself?

This is another example of your getting the information that someone would get doing a traditional suicide assessment protocol, but you are doing it in a very different order in that you have already established evidence of many things he did right already, and are organizing the session on what needs to happen next. And yet it seems you get the information you would need in order to assess safety.

CARL: Something told me that either he had to go, or I had to go. By him going, he would go back to jail, or prison, where he belongs.

INSOO: Yeah.

CARL: I mean, that's my brother, I love him, but he is a menace to society. And you know, he can't, you know, function with, you know, people, you know, out here, you know, trying to do good. But, do yeah, it's like that.

INSOO : So, obviously, he's going to be around. He's your brother.

CARL: Oh yeah, he's going to be around.

INSOO: So this is more . . . this is likely to happen again?

You are definitely not shying away from talking about the problem, and this may be important to point out because some readers may mistakenly think that SFBT therapists never talk about the problem or negative aspects of a situation.

CARL: Right, probably today, which I'm just—I just dread to go home.

INSOO: I can see that.

CARL: I hate going home.

INSOO: Of course. I understand that. So what do you need to do differently so that it doesn't happen again like last night?

It seems to function almost as a directive but it is much more gentle because it is in the form of a question.

CARL: I'm going to try to avoid him more. I mean, I usually do, but he'll either try to talk to me, or something like that. But the things he says to me, you know, is not like the conversation we're holding right now. It'll be something negative. Like my brother, he used to be out in a gang, and word has it he's still in a gang. He's a Blood and supposedly, me wearing blue all the time, but I'm wearing red. You know, I like all colors; you know, I don't discriminate with colors. They're just colors. I mean, why should somebody fight over another color that they hate? You know, with him, he hates me—he hates a little piece of me 'cause I like blue, and he doesn't like blue. So within our conversations, he'll tell me to—I'm not going to say on-camera—but he'll say like, you know, bring a profanity about, you know, the color blue and all that. And that red is, "red turns heads," meaning like, red is the spotlight and all that. But I mean, I like red, I like blue, I like every color . . .

INSOO: Yeah.

CARL: . . . but why are you hating one color?

INSOO: Yeah. So what will you . . . what do you have to do next time?

CARL: I'm going to . . .

INSOO: He's not going to change.

CARL: No, never.

INSOO: Yeah. Sounds like he's not likely to change . . .

CARL: Right.

INSOO: . . . anytime soon.

CARL: Right.

INSOO: So, what do you have to do next time so that this doesn't happen again like last night?

CARL: I really have to get out, I think.

INSOO: Get out?

CARL: I have to try to avoid him. If then we're around the house and I'm trying to avoid him, or he talks to me or something, that's my cue right there that I need to leave. I need to get away from there, 'cause each time I've stayed in that house and let it happen, I would always get beat up. I would always get hit with something. Like, we would fight with weapons.

INSOO: Wow.

CARL: I mean, it was like, chairs and ladders and lamps, anything that you could name, we broke tables, everything. My mom, she probably went through like, I don't know, about four different tables with us 'cause you know, it was that bad.

INSOO: Okay. So, first of all is not to tangle with your brother.

CARL: Right.

INSOO: Just walk away.

CARL: Right.

INSOO: Do you know at what point you need to walk away?

CARL: Not really.

INSOO: Not really?

CARL: I'm stuck. I just, like I told you earlier, I'm a reactor.

INSOO: Right.

CARL: I mean, if somebody—my mom told me, you know, "If somebody treats you with respect, do them the same, but if somebody treats you with disrespect, try to reason them out." But then again, if they just get to the point where they just you know, either scare you or you feel threatened—

INSOO: Or become violent?

CARL: Yeah, then, then, and just leads to your imagination, like from there.

INSOO: Yeah.

CARL: Like last night, that was just a straight-up reaction. I, you know, said everything there was out of the profanity book *[laughs]*, so.

> Do we acknowledge or pursue it if the client's nonverbal communication is markedly different from statements?
>
> We respond by asking more questions; however, we do not interpret, but accept what the client says.

INSOO: Right.

CARL: But I don't want it to happen again.

INSOO: So, what can best help you in a situation like that, like last night?

CARL: I mean, family talks to me. I mean, I get a lot of, you know, a lot of support from my family, well some of them. You know, some of them are negative.

INSOO: Who in your family?

> It is very important to get the details of what, where, who, when, how, and so on. The client's strength and resiliency show in small things they do, not in huge, heroic things they do.

CARL: Most of my cousins, really, 'cause you know, they've been through the same thing.

INSOO: With him?

CARL: No. With suicidal thoughts, or with their—well, kind of like him, with their brother also.

> I assumed that his cousins had similar encounters with his brother. But it turns out that his cousins also had suicidal episodes. It seems like he had a suicide support group in the family.

INSOO: Yeah, okay.

CARL: Excuse me. 'Cause he was, like, my brother.

INSOO: Yeah. Right. So, talking to them helps? Talking to your cousins helps?

CARL: Yeah, it helps a whole bunch. And that's where—

INSOO: Really?

CARL: Yeah.

INSOO: Well, good.

CARL: And that's where I stayed at last night. And I only got an hour of sleep, 'cause I stayed up 'til like five, and then I was like, "Okay, wake me up in an hour." Next thing you know, they drove me to school, and here I am.

INSOO: Wow.

CARL: I didn't care how late I was; I was only like, thirty minutes late, but I called in before I came, so. I ain't never going to miss a day of school ever again . . .

INSOO: Really.

CARL: . . . you know, or be late or something, for something.

INSOO: Right. So school is very helpful for you. Being in school is very helpful.

CARL: School is so important to me. It's a home, it's a second home.

INSOO: Wow.

CARL: Yeah.

INSOO: Okay. Right. So, explain to me again, what is the first thing you will do when you come into a situation like that with your brother or is it with other people in the family?

Wittgenstein reminds us that "the things that are most important for us are [often] hidden because of their simplicity and familiarity" and he says that frequently "one is unable to notice something—because it is always before one's eyes . . . and this means: we fail to be struck by what, once seen, is most striking and most powerful" (PI, #129).

CARL: It's normally with my brother.

INSOO: Normally with your brother?

CARL: In particular.

INSOO: Him in particular?

CARL: With other family, I can reason them out, or I can—

INSOO: You can manage.

CARL: Yeah, I can manage. But with him, it's a reaction.

INSOO: You don't know.

CARL: Yeah.

INSOO: You don't know. You're saying you always react.

CARL: Right.

INSOO: Okay. So, if you have to react, I guess you will have to walk away?

This question [I guess you will have to walk away] seems to reflect a stance helping Carl identify the details of his responses, thereby breaking them down to a series of many steps in a way that gives him much more control and a practical map of things he can do in the future to be safe, and yet you develop all of it solely with questions.

I suppose this is the closest I come to being directive, so that Carl can walk away with concrete steps he needs to remember. You will see later these three steps are revisited over and over.

CARL: Something like that.

INSOO: Something like that? Before you reach a point of having to react.

CARL: Yeah, but sometimes, like when a body is in a situation, it's steadfast, you know, it's, you know, in place. I usually listen to what he's telling me, and then it goes through my brain, and then whatever comes out, it comes out. And that's what I'm scared of, because sometimes you can say the wrong words to somebody.

INSOO: That's right.

CARL: That'll, you know . . .

INSOO: Trigger something.

CARL: But you know, yeah, in that kind of situation, it's unstoppable.

INSOO: Right.

CARL: Especially with him, he's just . . .

INSOO: Yeah.

CARL: I mean, there was a time where I was scared of him. I'm a little scared of him now, of what he kind of would do to me, but I'm mostly scared of what I'm going to do to him.

INSOO: Ah.

CARL: So, I'm trying to avoid that the best way I can.

INSOO: Wow, amazing, amazing. So what would be the first small sign that would tell you, "Uh-oh, I better walk away?"

CARL: The first sign . . .

INSOO: The first small sign that tells you, "This is a dangerous situation."

CARL: A small sign would be my heart pounding.

INSOO: Okay.

CARL: That happens all the time. If I'm arguing with somebody, my heart pounds and pounds. That's dangerous.

INSOO: So when you feel that . . .

CARL: Yeah.

INSOO: . . . you say, "This is time to get out."

CARL: Yeah, that's a warning sign.

INSOO: That's a warning sign.

CARL: But then, once stuff comes out of my mouth, my head starts to hurt. That's the other sign.

INSOO: Yeah.

CARL: That's the bad one, like, that's when the conflict comes in.

INSOO: Okay, so by the time your head starts to hurt, is that too late?

CARL: No.

INSOO: Or do you still have time?

CARL: I still have time.

INSOO: You still have time to walk away.

CARL: Like, last night, I actually hit my head and snapped out of it and said, "I'm going to cool off." So basically, I sort of got in control for the first time.

INSOO: Yes, you did.

CARL: This is the first time . . .

INSOO: Yes, you did.

CARL: . . . that I actually got in control.

INSOO: Yes, you did. Right. So, the heart pounding is the first sign.

CARL: The head hurting . . .

INSOO: The head hurts is the second sign. Something coming out of your mouth is the third sign.

CARL: And then, trying to avoid that, I try to either hit my head or try to snap out of it.

INSOO: Snap out of it.

CARL: Or try to go outside or something.

INSOO: What do you mean, hit your head?

CARL: As in, you know . . . you know, somebody try to snap, you know, slap somebody out of their, you know, coma or something.

INSOO: So, you go like that? *[Gestures as if hitting the side of her head.]*

CARL: Yeah, I'll go like that real, real hard and I'll just be—

INSOO: Real hard?

CARL: Real hard, and I'll say, "I'm going to go cool off."

INSOO: Okay, and that's a signal to you?

CARL: Right.

INSOO: So that's step three, it sounds like.

CARL: Yeah.

INSOO: Yeah.

CARL: In between.

INSOO: In between, right. So you have some time to walk out the door?

CARL: Exactly. But sometimes it doesn't work; this time it worked, but other times, it's just step one and two.

INSOO: Okay, all right. So which is safest? What step do you need to act if it is the safest? Step one, heart pounding, heart pounding, headache, or something coming out of your mouth?

CARL: Oh, it's my heart, all the time.

INSOO: The heart?

CARL: Your heart is your key to life, actually. I mean, if it beats harder, something is wrong, even if it's something good like adrenalin, like you're on a roller-coaster ride or something like that.

INSOO: You're right.

CARL: The heart pounding is, you know, you having fun or something like that. But the heart pounding when you're off in that type of situation, you should just, you know, leave, and I'm going to do that.

INSOO: Okay. That's a signal to you?

CARL: Yeah.

INSOO: "Uh-oh, danger is coming."

CARL: Right. I'll just get out then.

INSOO: Get out.

CARL: Instead of trying to listen to what he has to say.

INSOO: Right, right.

CARL: Yeah.

INSOO: Okay. How confident are you that you can do this? When your heart pounds, "Uh-oh, get out?"

This is an example of an assessment of safety in addition to finding out if more work needs to be done.

CARL: I'm most confident when words come out of my mouth.

INSOO: Oh, that's the sure sign?

What is your goal in asking this series of questions?

Most people describe reactions to violence as very impulsive, but in fact there are many steps. I want him to understand how it works in terms of how much time he has at each point. This creates a practical map he can use later when he needs it in real life. There are two main ways to do this and both involve questions: scaling and relational questions.

CARL: Yeah.

INSOO: Okay, so you still have some time?

CARL: I still have some time.

INSOO: Yeah, some time.

CARL: To break it.

INSOO: To break out of it.

CARL: But if I don't hit my head in time, something can go wrong.

INSOO: Yeah.

CARL: And I don't want that to happen.

INSOO: Okay. All right. So you have not, all these years, though, living with your brother, you have not actually hurt him, or hurt anybody?

CARL: No.

INSOO: No. You haven't.

CARL: I was the one being hurt. I mean, I tried to defend myself as best as I could, but . . .

INSOO: Right, but I meant, you have not been the one to start . . .

CARL: Oh no.

INSOO: . . . attacking someone?

CARL: No.

INSOO: It's usually him.

CARL: It's him, all the time.

This exchange gave further evidence that he does not instigate fights but indeed is "a reactor."

INSOO: Okay, Okay. All right. Okay, wow.

CARL: Yeah, I know what you're thinking. You're kind of like, well, what is this kid doing here? He seems kind of like a pretty nice guy, but he has all these problems. I usually think of that too, sometimes.

INSOO: Yeah? What is your answer then? What is your answer to yourself, when you ask that, when you say that to yourself? I wan't thinking that, but now that you mention it.

It would be very tempting to reassure him at this point, but again, it is much more powerful when it is a self-compliment out of his own assessment of himself that is more believable.

CARL: Now that I mention it?

INSOO: Yeah.

CARL: I don't know, I think as a person, you know, I'm very sincere. You know, I can cooperate.

INSOO: I believe you. I absolutely believe you.

CARL: I'm always willing to try anything if it, you know, leads to an answer or something.

INSOO: Yeah.

CARL: But, uh . . . yeah. The other thing . . . oh, I'm sorry, I messed up. Well, you know how your mind just wanders, but, uh . . .

INSOO: Yeah. So, when you ask that kind of question, "What is this kind of kid doing here?"

CARL: Oh yeah.

INSOO: What's your answer, what do you say to yourself?

CARL: Sometimes I say, "What am I doing?" That's the bad side. The good side is, "You're getting help," or "You're talking it out."

INSOO: Okay. Okay. And, you're saying, that's what helps, here in school?

CARL: Right.

INSOO: That's what you like about this school?

CARL: When I'm here I am so comfortable; I'm relaxed.

INSOO: You're calm?

CARL: I'm calm.

"Mere description is so difficult because one believes that one needs to fill out the facts to understand them. It is as if one saw a screen with scattered color-patches, and said: the way they are here, they are unintelligible; they only make sense when one completes them into a shape.—Whereas I want to say: Here is the whole. (If you complete it, you falsify it.)" (RPP1, #257).

INSOO: You're calm and this is your real self?

Once again, he is indicating that following your questions to elicit evidence of his competency, he now solidly identifies with himself as a competent person.

I knew the interview has achieved its function, that is, the client has a concrete plan of what he would need to do next time.

CARL: This is my self right here.

INSOO: Coming out.

CARL: Right here.

INSOO: In this school?

CARL: Right.

INSOO: Okay.

CARL: And then, today earlier with you and me with the discussion . . .

INSOO: Yes, that's you.

CARL: That's me.

INSOO: That's the real Carl?

CARL: Right.

"Since everything lies open to view there is nothing to explain" (PI, #126) at the conclusion of the conversation.

INSOO: I see. And you'd like to see more of those real Carls come out?

CARL: Sometimes.

INSOO: Well, those kind are very charming, very likeable and personable.

CARL: *[Laughs.]* Oh, man.

INSOO: Yes, you are? You are. And you know, you still have to go to Japan.

CARL: Oh, I am.

INSOO: Someday.

CARL: I will.

INSOO: Yeah. You're going to learn Japanese, you said.

CARL: Yeah, I'm going to try to save up. I took Japanese when I started seventh grade and eighth grade.

INSOO: Yeah?

CARL: And then it started getting kind of hard.

INSOO: Yes, it's getting really complicated.

CARL: Yeah, and my teacher's like, "Well, Carl, can you do it?" And I was like, "I have no idea." I got to high school, and I heard that they weren't having Japanese and I was just—I was so upset, so I just went through high school until my junior year. My teacher, Ms. Fuji, came and I was "Oh yes, I'm taking Japanese, all the way, I'm taking it." And I did so well up in that class. Every—well, the first semester, I had a 100 average, and the second was a 99 average 'cause I had one point off my exam. And that was it. So, yeah, I did pretty well in that class.

> Throughout this section, you are being such a wonderful audience for his competencies. This is part of the SFBT approach. These are what we work for, it seems, and such a pleasure to see this young man self-complimenting indirectly. What an honor to witness this!

INSOO: Japanese is a very difficult language.

CARL: Yeah. I like it, though. To me it's kind of easy in some way.

INSOO: Really?

CARL: Yeah.

INSOO: Do you speak . . . I mean, have you learned other languages besides Japanese?

CARL: I'm trying to work on my Spanish a little bit.

INSOO: Spanish?

CARL: But, I mean, I can read Spanish and speak it, but I can't really write it that well; like, how you spell this and that or the, you know, adjectives, and all that stuff, the complicated stuff. So I've been browsing at Swahili a little bit.

INSOO: My goodness.

CARL: And another thing is Arabic. Yeah, on my scholarship plan, well, whenever I took the SAT, they told me to put down the colleges that I wanted. First I put down ACC because that's my start right there, I figure. And then once I'm ready, I put down UT. I put down HT, and then I put down the University of Cairo in Egypt.

INSOO: Cairo? University of Cairo? Oh.

CARL: Yeah.

INSOO: Well, you have a long way to go, though, to learn enough to speak . . .

CARL: Yeah, Arabic.

INSOO: Yeah, Arabic. Well, ambitious young man.

CARL: Yeah, and the whole thing about the you know, the languages is because I want, you know, I want to travel. I ain't never been out of Texas, ever.

INSOO: Oh.

CARL: I mean, I've been city to city; like, I've been to Waco, something like that, or Houston a couple of times, but I haven't been out.

INSOO: Oh, so you want to really broaden your experience?

CARL: I want to just travel.

INSOO: Travel.

CARL: And hope I get there with my, you know, abilities that I'm going to ACC for.

INSOO: Yeah, yeah.

CARL: I'm majoring in Performing and Song Writing. So hopefully I can.

INSOO: Wonderful. Wonderful. Wow. So what do you have to keep your eye on this side of you? Just keep your eye on this side.

CARL: Stay positive all the time.

INSOO: Okay.

CARL: Do something happy every day. I mean, some people would want to go a day or two or a week without, you know, not laughing or not, you know, not, enjoying themselves. I want to enjoy myself every day if I have to. If there's something on, you know, like a show that makes me laugh, like *American Idol [laughs],* or something like that, you know, I'll watch that, you know, cheer me up. You need something—I mean for me to be focused, I need to be, you know, balanced out. You know, I need to have my laughs here; I need to have, you know, a little quiet, just a little bit, and then I have to have my dream up there, concentrate on my dream.

> Here Carl is reminding himself to be happy, perhaps to wear his "happy face" that he talked about earlier. This is quite a useful way of going about daily life.

INSOO: Okay, so you know exactly what you need.

CARL: Yup, and it's all here, really.

INSOO: It's all here, in school, in this school.

CARL: Right.

INSOO: Wonderful. Okay, all right. So, you will continue to talk with your counselor about this, right?

CARL: Right. Oh yeah, as a matter of fact, after we leave here, I have to talk to him.

INSOO: Okay.

CARL: About earlier that I was talking about, you know, when I hurt myself. I actually broke my contract because according to the—in the MHMR, they call it that—"Mental Health, Mental Resources" or whatever . . . which, I actually told my mom to go ahead and put me in, you know, something like that, for me to get counseling for my, you know, suicidal thoughts and depression and all that. I signed a contract saying that I wouldn't hurt myself or anybody else, and I broke it. And I don't know what's going to happen after that, but hopefully it'll be a warning 'cause the possibilities are if I break it, then they'll have to put me off in a place for a while, and I don't want that . . . at all. You know, I'll tell them, I'll go to school all day if I have to, or try to stay with somebody, try to get my own place, but anything but staying off in a place like that.

INSOO: Right, so it's very clear about what you don't want.

CARL: Right.

INSOO: Yeah. Okay. All right. So I would suggest that you continue talking with the counselors here.

CARL: Yeah, Mr. Licce.

INSOO: Yeah, Mr. Licce.

CARL: Um, Mr. Licce, he's been there for . . . I don't know, he's been there a great deal. Top one, A.

INSOO: Yeah. All right. You are a remarkable young man.

CARL: Thank you. And you're a remarkable . . . young woman.

INSOO: *[Laughs.]* Old lady! Old lady!

CARL: Young woman, young woman! *[Laughs.]*

INSOO: Tell the truth. I appreciate it very much, this chance to talk to you. And you've been so helpful, during this morning.

CARL: Yeah.

INSOO: Yeah. You're like a star. You are the star of the whole group.

CARL: No.

INSOO: *[Laughs.]* You are so funny.

CARL: *[Laughs.]* Nah.

INSOO: And I'm going to give you "A" for this talking to me. You'll finally get your A. Not F but finally get your A. Do you want me to write it down for you?

CARL: No, I got it, I got it.

INSOO: You got it? You got it in your mind?

CARL: Yeah.

INSOO: Right. Okay. All right, Carl.

CARL: And I hope to see you in Japan in July, hopefully.

INSOO: Wonderful. I enjoyed talking to you very much.

CARL: *[Japanese.]*

INSOO: *[Japanese.]* Okay, good.

Chapter 8

Private Experience and the Verb "To Be"

Even when working with problems involving such apparently internal, private experiences as emotional states, SFBT therapists typically use outward criteria (scales and observable behaviors designated by the client). Following Wittgenstein's practice of focusing on external rather than internal criteria to signify change is a radical departure, not just from Freud, but from Western philosophical traditions.

The traditional view, Cartesianism for example, is based upon a radical disjunction between inside and outside (mind and body). In this view, mental and emotional states and processes are seen to be radically private and only the individual has access to them; they are hidden from other people. Thus, each individual person is encapsulated within his own ideas and emotions. According to this traditional model,

> one has direct access to his or her own ideas, feelings and sensations, but no direct access to anything external, i.e., to the material world or to the minds of others. Such access, if possible at all, is at best inferential and at most probable. In one's own case certainty about one's ideas and feelings is possible because no inference is required (Stroll, 2002, p. 117).

Wittgenstein argues against this perspective in many different ways:

> The essential thing about private experience is really not that each person possesses his own exemplar, but that nobody knows whether other people also have this or something else. The assumption would thus be possible—though unverifiable—that one section of mankind had one sensation of red, another section another (PI, #272).

What is called his "private language argument" involves one of his "mind experiments" which I (SdS) hope to simplify without losing his primary argument. Suppose that my friend Max experienced a private, inner sensation, one that he had never experienced before and for which he had no name. So Max wrote the letter "S" on a piece of paper to remind himself of this unique sensation. When the sensation happened again, he wrote another "S" on the piece of paper. The sensation recurred many times and Max continued marking "S" each time until he filled a small notebook. This notebook is sort of a ledger documenting the existence of Max's private, inner "S" experiences. Now, let's suppose that Max decides to show you his ledger, explaining that he wants to share his "S" experience with you. You carefully look and see page after page filled with strings of "S's." You, of course, want to make some sense of this in order to imagine what "S" must feel like and to share Max's experience with him.

But this is a radically private and fully internal sensation, one that only Max has had and which is not marked by any external signs other than "S." How can you make sense of it? All you know is that Max calls it "S." How can you imagine what "S" feels like, since it is internal? How would you know when Max is feeling an "S" sensation in your presence, since this experience has no outward manifestations? How would you know if you had an "S" experience of your own? Is it possible you already did? Might you have a private, inner experience that you think is the same as Max's "S" sensation but really is not?

These are the kinds of questions you might reasonably ask about Max's "S" experiences and ledger. If you actually asked these questions of Max, then you would have to deal with the responses, to try and make some sense of them. All of your questions and the difficulty Max has in answering them suggest to Max that he really has no firm basis for declaring that all of these sensations that he baptized as "S's" are the same. Might some be baptized "R" and others "T"? Like you, Max has no external or independent sources for verifying his impressions and memory of the sensations, or for changing his designation of them as all "S's." Given these difficulties, it would be reasonable for you and Max to decide that, despite your best efforts, you cannot share Max's "S" experience and he cannot ever be certain that all of the sensations were really "S's."

Without outward criteria, it makes no difference whether or not all the "S's" are the same or whether each one was completely different from all the others. No certainty is possible here. Furthermore, it makes no difference whether or not Max ever really had these experiences. That is, nothing changes for you if Max did not have these experiences but just says he did. Lacking outward criteria, there is nothing to go on here.

Thus, in Wittgenstein's view, the individual does not have special, private knowledge about his or her own inner states and processes. In order for us to talk about, make sense of, and perhaps define, these inner processes, we need outward criteria that can be referenced by and shared with others.

> Wittgenstein also questions the assumption which unites dualism, materialism, and behaviorism, namely that first-person present tense psychological utterances are descriptions or reports—if not of a soul, then of the brain or behavior. He claims that in fact they are typically *avowals*, expressions of the inner which are in some respects analogous to natural reactions, gestures, grimaces, etc. (Glock, 1996, pp. 175-176).

The uniform appearance of words such as "depression," "happy," "angry," and "hope" encourages us to assume that the words refer to an entity about which we can generalize. We often treat uniform-appearing words as if the words carry halos of meaning that they retain regardless of context. We often assume that words that refer to presumably inner, private experiences operate in the same way as words that refer to publicly observable objects.

Compare → I feel happy. / He feels happy.

The criteria we might use for saying "He feels happy" are rather commonplace and include smiles, laughs, sparkling eyes, etc. Do I look for criteria in order to say "I am happy"? Where do I feel happy? In my face? Clearly not. I simply have some sort of sensation that I call "happy." This is not a matter of knowledge; it is just an exclamation.

When I say "He feels happy," there is always some chance that he might deny this. But, when I say "I feel happy," there is no chance that I might be wrong about this. (I might, of course, be lying.) Interestingly, without the possibility of being wrong, I also cannot be right.

Compare → I feel angry. / He feels angry.
I feel anxious. / He feels anxious.

He is scowling and therefore we say "He feels angry" and he is rapidly pacing back and forth and therefore we say "He feels anxious." If we ask him, he will either confirm or disconfirm our judgment. Again, it is not as if we observe ourselves and see ourselves scowling or pacing back and forth and thus come to a conclusion about how we feel. Rather, both "I feel angry" and "I feel anxious" are just exclamations about which I can be neither right nor wrong. That is, both are more similar to "Ouch" than they are to statements of knowledge or reports on our inner states.

Compare → I feel like a good cook. / He feels like a good cook.

There are only certain, specific contexts in which "I feel like a good cook" that are primarily limited to observing people eat what I cooked. When they ask for seconds without more being offered, or when the dish that should be for six to eight is barely enough for five people, or when they ask for the recipe, then "I feel like a good cook." There may be other times, such as when I am cooking something in which I have a lot of confidence, but that's only once in a while. Usually I do not feel like a good cook; I have other types of feelings. I am quite sure that when "I feel like a good cook" in the situations listed above, other people will see signs that might lead them to say "He feels like a good cook," but that is not a normal way to talk about it; they would be much more likely to say "He feels good." If the cooking is talked about at all, the other people will usually say something such as "He is a good cook," which is altogether different.

Compare → He is a good cook. / I feel like a good cook. / I am a good cook.

The statement "I feel like a good cook" is situational and rather fleeting. On the other hand, because of the verb "to be," the statement "I am a good cook" is a statement about me rather than an avowal about how I feel. In other words, "I am a good cook" no matter what I am doing; even when I am writing or walking in the park I can say "I am a good cook." The switch in verbs from "to feel" to "to be" takes us from observations that could easily be expanded to include the context to talking about something that is a permanent, enduring attribute of the individual. Once the shift is made, the sentence is no longer limited to the context of watching people eat what I have cooked. The sentence is no longer about cooking and feeling that it is a job well done but rather it is now about me. Switching from "to feel" to "to be" removes the context, and the experience of pleasure (or anger or anxiety or happiness) disappears.

There is, of course, a rather striking difference between "He is a good cook" and "I am a good cook." My use of the words "I am" leads you to seek verification and there are cues, criteria available to you. This data would allow you as an observer to be able to say "He is a good cook." No problem. Many people I've cooked for can (and most do) say "He is a good cook." However, my saying "I am a good cook" may or may not be necessarily based on some sort of criteria.

> How should we counter someone who told us that with him understanding was an inner process?—How should we counter him if he said that with him knowing how to play chess was an inner process?—We should say that when we want to know if he can play chess we aren't interested in anything that goes on inside him.—And if he replies that this is in fact just what we are interested in, that is, we are interested in whether he can play chess—then we shall have to draw his attention to the criteria which would demonstrate his capacity, and on the other hand to the criteria for the "inner states" (PI, #181).

THE VERB "TO BE"

Let's look further at the verb "to be."

> In the language of everyday life it very often happens that the same word signifies in two different ways—and therefore belongs to two different symbols . . . Thus the word "is" appears as the copula, as the sign of equality, and as the expression of existence . . . (T, #3.323). Thus there easily arise the most fundamental confusions (of which the whole of philosophy is full) (T, #3.324).

Compare → I am male. / He is a male.
I am an American. / He is an American.
I am a good cook. / He is a good cook.

I can say that "I am a male," "I am an American," "I am a good cook," because I am certain that I am a male, an American, and a good cook. But these are not really statements of knowledge and may or may not be based on some empirical criteria. Being a male, an American, and a good cook are all enduring or permanent attributes, facts of life for me. Even though now and then my cooking will be a disaster, as I see it, these beliefs are not subject to change. As Wittgenstein put it: "He has got to know that he knows: for knowing is a state of his own mind; he cannot be in doubt or error about it" (Z, #408).

The situation changes when we shift from the first person present to the third person present. Again, my use of the words "I am" leads you to seek verification and there are cues, criteria available to you. This allows you as an observer to be able to say "He is a male," "He is an American." No problem. Insoo and other people I've cooked for can (and most do) say "He is a good cook." Wittgenstein points out an important distinction here:

> Psychological verbs [are] characterized by the fact that the third person of the present is to be verified by observation, the first person not. Sentences in the third person of the present: *information*. In the first person present: *expression* [Emphasis added]. (Z, #472)

Compare → I am a male. / He is a male.
I am an American. / He is an American.
I am a good cook. / He is a good cook.
I am a schizophrenic. / He is a schizophrenic.

What happens in the fourth pair of sentences? Remember the DSM and the long tradition of diagnosis in psychiatry. The form of the verb "to be" is the same in all four first person present verbs (I am an X) and it is also the same in each of the third person present verbs (He is an X). The "is" in all four sentences using the third person singular involves the same grammatical form of identity (2 x 2 *is* 4). This is very seductive, leading us to automatically process the sentences in the same way and it leads us inevitably to the conclusion that schizophrenia is similar to being male, an

American, and a good cook: All four are seen as or implicitly understood as permanent and enduring attributes of the individual.

Compare → 2 x 2 is 4. / He = schizophrenic.
The rose is red. / Rose ≠ red.

The grammar of the "is" in sentence #2 here is different from the "is" in sentence #1. The verb "is" here is something that bonds two different things together, rose and red, rather than the sign of existence or identity. In other words, red is not identical with rose, nor is rose identical with red. Some roses are white, some yellow, etc.

Our grammar leads us, naturally, to the conclusion that schizophrenia is incurable: once a schizophrenic, always a schizophrenic. We do not need psychiatry or even theory for this, just grammar.

Compare → I am an alcoholic. / He is an alcoholic.

What happens here? Evidently AA, like psychiatry (at least in the case of schizophrenia), is seduced by the verb "to be" into believing that being an alcoholic is a steady state, something permanent. This leads to the idea that in spite of 30 years without a drink, he is still an alcoholic! The "is" within this mythology is in fact so strong that probably no empirical evidence will influence AA or the diagnostic language-game. Cure is impossible.

Compare → I am an anorexic. / She is an anorexic.

And here? The Anti-Anorexia League seems to have been seduced by the grammar of "to be." From their perspective, the "cure" for anorexia involves a lifelong fight against anorexia that "proves" that the "is" does indeed stand for the equal sign: She = anorexic. Thus, while starving herself (suffering from anorexia), anorexia is the problem. After the "cure," anorexia remains the problem in the form of "anti-anorexia." (In Logic, as Wittgenstein pointed out, the "p" in the statements "p" and "not-p" must stand for the same thing.)

* * *

Compare → I feel better. / I am better.
You feel better. / You are better.
He feels better. / He is better.

When asked, as therapy progresses, clients usually report "feeling better." Because of the transitory nature of the verb "to feel," the therapist will look at the context around this exclamation and as the description or depiction becomes richer and fuller, he or she can begin to shift to the verb "to be" in order to take advantage of its grammar. In other words, at some point, through the use of scales and descriptions of the various numbers on the scale and other descriptions of the client's daily life, the "evidence" will build to the point that the therapist can say something like: "Wow! It is clear that you are better." This then logically leads to questions about how the client is going to maintain the improvement.

* * *

How does this work with other psychiatric diagnostic categories? As Wittgenstein puts it: "Anything your reader can do for himself leave to him" (CV, p. 77e).

* * *

Let's look briefly at the verb "to think."

> The tangled use of "think" . . . As if the word "violin" referred not only to the instrument, but sometimes to the violinist, the violin part, the sound, or even the playing of the violin (RPP2, #730).

In seminars and workshops, after I (SdS) have demonstrated interviewing a client (or shown a videotape of an interview), I am often asked: "What were you thinking when . . ." at some particular point(s) during the interview, which the questioner then goes on to describe. My usual answer: "Nothing apart from what you have seen and heard" satisfies me, but clearly not the questioner. As Wittgenstein puts it:

> I can know what the other person is thinking, not what I am thinking. It is correct to say "I know what you're thinking," wrong to say "I know what I'm thinking." [An entire cloud of philosophy condenses to one droplet of grammar.] (PI, p. 222)

The questioner sees and hears what both the client and I did immediately before the questioned point in the interview—for example, the asking of the miracle question. As a result of many years of practice I now ask the miracle question automatically, without *thinking* in the sense of that term that the questioner is using. It is not a matter of saying to myself "Aha, now is the time," nor it is a matter of intuition. Rather, it is a result of training. An observer, of course, could carefully watch many, many sessions that include the therapist's asking the miracle question and figure out some rules that seem to hold. The rules might deal with something like this: In the greatest majority of cases, before the miracle question is asked, the client has talked about what kind of results he or she might want from therapy and thus indirectly at least has told the therapist that he or she believes change is possible. Frequently the client will have told the therapist about exceptions of some sort that will have allowed the therapist to compliment the client in some way. Also, the client will usually have at least sketched his or her daily life so that the context of the response to the miracle question will make some sense because it fits within an already described context.

In some ways I want to say that I do not know when to ask the miracle question, I just do it. This is somewhat similar to the following: When driving I shift appropriately from second to third or from third to second without thinking about it at all. It is simply a matter of training and experience. Wittgenstein says it well: "He 'thinks' when, in a definite kind of way, he perfects a method he has" (Z, #104). Of course, when to ask the miracle question is difficult to know without a lot of practice and observation. Therefore the questioner's query is entirely reasonable. However, the questioner's question treats thinking as if it were some sort of separate, simultaneous activity that takes place while the conversation is going on.

> If a normal human is holding a normal conversation under such and such normal circumstances, and I were asked what distinguishes thinking from not-thinking in such a case—I should not know what answer to give. And I could certainly not say that the difference lay in something that goes on or fails to go on while he is speaking (RPP2, #248).

The questioner indeed treats thinking as a separate, simultaneous, and parallel activity that occurs while the conversation goes on. However, thinking is not behavior. Interestingly, as we observe session after session it becomes clear that thinking can most easily be described as the conversation itself. The confusion arises because

> the existence of the words denoting (bodily) activities, such as writing, speaking, etc., makes us look for an activity, different from these but analogous to them, corresponding to the word "thinking." When words in our ordinary language have prima facie analogous grammar we are inclined to try to interpret them analogously; i.e., we try to make the analogy hold throughout (BBB, p. 7).

Wittgenstein frequently pointed out the difficulties involved with the concept of "thinking" and suggested that a lot of trouble was created by philosophers who spoke about thinking as some sort of activity that occurs inside a person's head, thus making it into something occult and mysterious. Indeed, "'the concept of thinking' is formed on the model of a kind of imaginary auxiliary activity" (Z, #106).

> We know what "studying" or "finding out" about something is like—say, studying the workings of a machine or the anatomy of the body. So we propose to "study" or "find out about" thinking, about the mind. And now things become very puzzling indeed; we find ourselves deeply confused about the "mechanism" here and must propose a very peculiar, "occult" mechanism. We use the same words, the same form of expression, to describe two projects, and

> are misled into seeing them as more alike than they really are (Staten, 1984, p. 77).

Does the questioner in the seminar believe that I consult a rule book that is in my head? Yes, that's clear. This is exactly what the questioner seems to believe. However, I got to know how to do therapy by learning how to do therapy. In this way, at least, doing therapy is similar to driving a car; both are the result of training and practice. Therefore, when I drive, I follow "one-way" arrows automatically. In either case, what I do can be described as obeying the rules. However, I do not consciously follow the rules.

> "Obeying a rule" is a practice. And to think one is obeying a rule is not to obey a rule. Hence it is not possible to obey a rule "privately": otherwise thinking one was obeying a rule would be the same as obeying it (PI, #202).

Clearly there is a certain amount of predictability to therapy sessions, and the observer might refer to my behaving as if I am obeying the rules. But, as Wittgenstein puts it: "When I obey a rule, I do not choose. I obey the rule blindly" (PI, #219). In other words, in employing a rule I have mastered, I act as a matter of course.

We cannot separate thinking from the activity. During the interview, what I was "thinking" is clear and obvious based on close observation of the conversation itself. It is right there on the surface of the conversation—there is nothing hidden, nothing going on that cannot be heard and seen. (This is similar to asking a chess player about his chess thoughts while he is playing chess. What matters here is what is taking place on the chess board. His thoughts are shown by the moves he makes publicly on the board and not something mysterious only the chess player is aware of.)

"We cannot separate his 'thinking' from his work. For thinking is not an accompaniment of . . . thoughtful speech" (Z, #101). If I were to be "thinking," i.e., talking to myself about what to do next, then I would be unable to hear what the client was saying. I would be much too busy listening to myself and thus unable to respond in useful ways. If "thinking" were this sort of auxiliary activity, then meaningful conversation would be impossible; we would be too busy to engage.

* * *

> Don't see it as a matter of course, but as something very worthy of note, that the verbs "believe," "hope," "wish," "intend" and so on ["think"], exhibit all the grammatical forms that are also possessed by "eat," "talk," "cut" (RPP1).

Chapter 9

SFBT and Emotions

> The events of the future cannot be inferred from those of the present. The belief in the causal nexus is a superstition.
>
> —Wittgenstein (T, #5.1361).

* * *

Over the years, SFBT has frequently been criticized for how the approach "deals with emotions" and even, sometimes, for "ignoring the emotions." Somehow or other, some therapists got the idea that the apparent focusing on behavior means that SFBT "ignores emotions" or "excludes emotions." This criticism is, of course, based on the traditional ways both philosophy and psychology—and thus psycho-therapy—have viewed "emotions and feelings." Traditionally, emotions and feelings were seen by philosophy and psychology as inner states or forces that are depicted as intimately, and frequently causally, related to the kinds of problems therapists treat. This individualistic and linear, causal point of view privileges the subjective over the public and/or social as the starting place for our understanding of emotions and feelings. Thus, the individual is seen to have a special, infallible knowledge of his or her own inner states and forces. This view is fundamental to traditional psychology and psychiatry.

Wittgenstein sees emotions in a very different way. For instance, he would point to the context in which an individual experienced the emotion. He would remind us that in our ordinary use of words such as "anger," "fear," "anxiety," "better," "depressed," etc., other people are involved and whatever happened both before and after has something to do with the emotion we felt. In other words, the emotion—"anger," "better," "depressed," etc.—cannot be understood when it is cut off from the context that is its home; doing so makes the emotion into something mysterious and separate from everyday life.

Of course, as Wittgenstein would point out, this is something we already know, but the traditional worldview (inevitably based in large part on traditional philosophy and psychology) confuses us and gives us the urge to want to dig deeper and see what lies behind and beneath, to understand the essence of "feeling better" or "anger." We automatically forget the context of everyday life and are puzzled. Thus Wittgenstein saw his job—at least in part—as providing us with reminders of what we already know.

For Wittgenstein, any and all inner processes and states, such as feeling angry, feeling better, thinking, etc., are connected to and—at least in part—defined by some outside context. If an individual says "I feel depressed," this is an expression of his emotional or feeling state and is similar to an exclamation such as "ouch." It is not an empirical statement. It is not as if the individual were reporting on a personal observation of himself or herself. It is not a statement of knowledge. Since the first person present is not a report about something the individual knows about himself or herself but is just an expression, the individual cannot be wrong about it. Of course, since he or she cannot be wrong, he or she also cannot be right. It is just an exclamation. However, when we say, for example, "He is depressed," we are reporting on our observations—which again points to the context: We see him behaving in ways similar to how we saw other people behave who said they were depressed. Of course we could be wrong and only he can confirm or disconfirm our observation.

Wittgenstein's way of describing things reminds us to observe what is going on and reminds us to look at everyday life—including language as it is actually used—as the home of our concepts and descriptions. It is these descriptions of everyday life that replace the explanations and theories of traditional philosophy and psychology.

As I see it—Wittgenstein puts this nicely and clearly—any " 'inner process' [such as feelings of anger] stands in need of outward criteria" (PI, #580) and furthermore, he says, emotions are only important because of the context in which they arise (PI, p. 188).

An interesting problem develops here, however. As Wittgenstein puts it:

> The first step is the one that altogether escapes notice. We talk of [inner] processes and states and leave their nature undecided. Sometime perhaps we shall know more about them—we think. But that is just what commits us to a particular way of looking at the matter. For we have a definite concept of what it means to learn to know a process better. (The decisive movement in the conjuring trick has been made, and it was the very one we thought quite innocent.)—And now the analogy which was to make us understand our thoughts falls to pieces. So we have to deny the yet uncomprehended process in the yet unexplored medium. And now it looks as if we had denied [inner] process. And naturally we don't want to deny [inner processes, i.e., emotions] (PI, #308).

Thus, since inner processes are hidden from view, SFBT is often misunderstood as ignoring and/or denying emotions because we focus on the outer, visible criteria (behavior). Therefore, SFBT is further misunderstood as some sort of behaviorism. "The impression that we wanted to deny something arises from our setting our faces against the picture of the 'inner process'" (PI, #305) which we cannot see. "What we deny is that the picture of the inner process give us the correct idea of the use of the word" (PI, #305) or concept of "emotions."

* * *

For example, after the therapist and client have explored the client's description of the day-after-the-miracle, the therapist will usually ask a scaling question.

THERAPIST: Now, on a scale from "0" to "10" with "10" standing for how things are the day after the miracle . . .

CLIENT: Okay . . .

THERAPIST: . . . and "0"—an arbitrary starting point—standing for how things were when you arranged for this appointment . . .

CLIENT: Okay . . .

THERAPIST: Where are things now between "0" and "10"?

CLIENT: I'd have to say "3."

What are they talking about in this exchange? Both seem to know what they are talking about.

THERAPIST: So, what are the differences between "0" and "3"?

CLIENT: Well, at "0" I felt hopeless, really down and had to force myself to get out of bed . . .

THERAPIST: And at "3"?

CLIENT: I can see some hope . . . I'm more willing to do things that at "0" I would have had to force myself to do.

THERAPIST: What other differences would your best friend notice?

CLIENT: I'm able to smile sometimes.

At this point it is somewhat clearer that "10," "3" and "0" stand for—are shorthand or code words for—the client's inner states, i.e., feelings and emotions that the client is able now to more fully describe, sometimes in observable, behavioral terms. Scales thus are used to develop and describe the outward parts of a change in feelings.

THERAPIST: So, what would you and your best friend be doing when you are smiling sometimes?

CLIENT: We'd probably be sitting in a café having coffee—which is something we've not done lately because I just simply felt too damn down to bother.

THERAPIST: So, just getting together would be different when you got to "3"?

CLIENT: Yeah, particularly if I initiated it . . . That might even be a "4"!

THERAPIST: This would be a sign to your friend that you've changed, feel better?

CLIENT: Yeah, she'd know immediately—if I called—that I was feeling better.

THERAPIST: And how would she react?

CLIENT: She'd be pleased.

THERAPIST: And you'd be pleased that she's pleased . . .

CLIENT: Yeah, certainly . . .

THERAPIST: So, as a result, what would you two do?

CLIENT: Probably both have a dessert which neither of us should have *[laughs]*.

Clearly, the therapist and the client are talking about the outward signs and contexts of the client's change, i.e., feeling better. The client in fact introduced the next step of going from "3" to "4," a further improvement in how she feels.

Talking about having coffee and perhaps dessert in a café—when both women are feeling pleased and smiling—sometimes situates "feeling better" in its home base: everyday life. The next time she sees her friend she is likely to remember this bit of conversation and smile, which might prompt a smile in return. This might suggest to the client that she really does feel better. (They might even have the forbidden dessert and enjoy it.)

* * *

Of course, many times clients naturally talk about how they want other people to change. Since we are talking about situations and contexts as well as interactions, scales can be quite useful.

THERAPIST: So, "10" stands for you have as much confidence as anybody can have about anything that you'll remain abstinent and "0" stands for the opposite; where are you now?

CLIENT: "10."

THERAPIST: And where would you say your wife would say she is—if she were here?

CLIENT: "3"—Of course, that's just a guess . . .

THERAPIST: Sure, but you know her pretty well . . . How would she know that she's gone up from "3" to "4"?

CLIENT: It's a matter of trust, you see. It will take some time.

THERAPIST: Naturally; how long perhaps?

CLIENT: At least a month or two.

THERAPIST: How will she show you more trust, from "3" to "4"?

CLIENT: She probably won't. She's rather pissed with me, you see, and she keeps her distance.

THERAPIST: So, where on the same scale will she be when she shows you she's less pissed and more trustful?

CLIENT: At least "6" or perhaps even "7"?

THERAPIST: What will she do?

CLIENT: Perhaps she'd get up and make me a cooked breakfast—fried eggs, bacon, that sort of thing.

THERAPIST: Will that be a big or a small surprise?

CLIENT: Gigantic! *[Laughs.]* Might even be a miracle.

THERAPIST: So what will you do?

CLIENT: I'd give her a great big hug.

THERAPIST: Before or after eating?

CLIENT: Before . . .

The conversation moves back and forth between context, behavior, and feeling states, allowing the client to imagine the situation in which he and his wife are feeling significantly better about each other. Therefore, "feeling better" is not just some vague inner event or process, but is talked about in its normal, natural context, its home base. This is where the better feelings are wanted and significant to the client (and his wife).

EMOTIONS IN CONTEXT

Let us take a look at a very common type of sentence that is frequently used by all of us. Let's imagine a client says:

→ I yelled at her because I was angry. ←

What kind of work does this sentence do? Simply put, it might lead us to abstract the "angry" feeling from the context in which it happened, that is, we might wonder about why the client was angry. If he were to say that this is a frequent occurrence, we might then begin to wonder about his ability to control or manage his anger. Thus, the idea that the anger caused the yelling becomes confirmed and the anger becomes the problem upon which we focus in the traditional way.

If we had enlarged this picture and looked into what came before and what came after, how would the anger add to our understanding of the situation? Or, does the anger accidentally serve to hide the context, to remove both him and her from the picture, to focus our attention on his anger rather than on the interaction?

Removed from the context, he can only see himself and the trouble resulting from his yelling at her. Without a before or an after, he can say that she, of course, had nothing to do with it. (And, of course, she can say the same thing.) Without the context, his yelling is problematic but he has a ready excuse: his anger. He creates himself as a victim of his anger. Now, of course, the next step is to search for the "cause" of the anger itself, removing things further and further from the interaction between them and the context in which it happens. Both of them are off the hook; neither is responsible. Whatever happened, the anger is responsible. It is as if he is saying: The devil made me do it. (And thus "anger management groups" develop.)

My focus instead is first on the context in which the angry feeling happened. What happened before he yelled at her? What happened after? When and where did this happen? Although the angry feeling might not ever be mentioned again by name, talking about what happened before, during, and after the yelling certainly deals with the context, which is the outside part of the anger. Is it not clear that this approach deals with the client's emotions (inner and outer)? Is it not also clear that this approach may lead to changes in how he deals with her and/or how she deals with him, which might lead to his yelling at her less frequently and also to his feeling angry less often in this particular context? Of course this social, interactional approach is not the same as the traditional, individualistic approach. (I suspect this is what the critics mean by their criticism—SFBT does not deal with "emotions" in the same way(s) as other approaches. This is obviously true regardless of what particular problem is looked at.)

Furthermore, I am most interested in any kind of "exceptions." I wonder about any times when he was angry and did not yell at her, and other times, in different contexts, when he was angry and did not yell. What are the differences between times when he yelled and times when he did not? I also am interested in times when the context was similar and he was not angry. Are there times when he yelled but was not angry? All these are ways of dealing with anger that keep the emotion within its natural, contextual home of everyday life. (Of course this is not the traditional way, but this is clearly not ignoring the emotions.)

I focus on what he wants to be different when he is feeling better, whether or not that is obviously related to either being angry or yelling. It seems to me that talking about what he is doing when he is feeling better elicits more "better feelings" and the more details about the context he can describe, the easier it will be for him to remember how good "feeling better" feels. Plus, when significant other people see him "feeling better" i.e., doing something different, i.e., not showing his anger (the outside which is all they can know about) they will react in ways that serve to reinforce and help him remember his better feelings (inside).

Clearly, then, SFBT deals with emotions in ways that are not similar to the ways emotions are dealt with traditionally. But this does not mean that "emotions" are either ignored or minimized. Rather, the approach focuses on the outside, observable factors and context that define emotions. Furthermore, the approach helps clients focus on the hard work of remembering "better" feelings by helping to keep these feelings connected to the contexts that are their home in everyday life.

SFBT does not view emotions as problems to be solved but rather views them as some of the many resources that clients have for constructing something "better." In other words, helping clients construct situations where they "feel better" and where they can remember that they feel better is one part of successfully constructing and "reinforcing" solutions. By paying attention to the context in which emotions happen, SFBT keeps them in their proper home, which is the client's everyday life, rather than making them an esoteric, mysterious phenomenon inside of the individual. Thus, other people who are involved in the client's everyday life help to, by accident, reinforce the changes they observe and participate in naturally and normally. This bridges the gulf clients in traditional therapies often experience as a result of the discrepancy between awareness of resourses in the therapy room and lack thereof in everyday life.

Let's take another look at:

→ I yelled at her because I was angry. ←

Does this mean that he thinks or believes that anger caused him to yell? Or, rather, is he giving anger as a justification (or a reason) for his yelling? The idea that his anger caused his yelling is a hypothesis and this

> "hypothesis is well-founded if one has had a number of experiences which, roughly speaking, agree in showing that your action is the regular sequel of certain conditions which we then call causes of the action" (BBB, p. 15).

The question here is whether or not a prediction can be made with any confidence that yelling will more often than not result from his being angry. However, it is a different situation when we want to know the reason he had for yelling because

> "no number of agreeing experiences is necessary, and the statement of your reason is not a hypothesis" (BBB, p. 15).

That is to say, for anger to be considered the cause of yelling, it would have to be shown that in a sufficient number of instances anger is regularly followed by yelling. (Of course, now and then he could be angry without that being followed by yelling.) On the other hand, a reason is characterized by his recognizing and accepting it as such: It seems perfectly reasonable to him that his anger was the reason he yelled at her. If he had not been angry there would not have been any reason to yell.

Shifting from the first person to the third:

→ He yelled at her because he was angry. ←

As long as the speaker recognizes and accepts that the anger was the reason for his yelling at her, then the observer can be comfortable with this attribution of anger as a reason. But the anger cannot be the reason for the yelling if he does not recognize and accept it as such. The fact that he may be unaware of a fair number of the reasons for his yelling does not change the reasons into causes or hypotheses.

> What he is unaware of in such a case are precisely reasons, not causes . . . Freud treats the reason for an action like a cause by supposing that it can be conjectured by a scientific sort of procedure and confirmed in the end by the acquiescence of the subject, who recognizes it as having indeed been his reason; and he treats the cause like a reason by supposing that the causes he seeks can be known in the second way, which has nothing to do with the way causal hypotheses are verified in an experimental science (Bouveresse, 1995, p. 72).

* * *

From Wittgenstein's perspective, Freud confused reason and cause, which led to an "abominable mess" that continues to this day.

> People who are constantly asking 'why' are like tourists who stand in front of a building reading [a tourists' guide] and are so busy reading the history of its construction, etc., that they are prevented from seeing the building (CV, p. 40e).

Wittgenstein drew a distinction between reasons and causes that is at odds with the traditional, causal conception of the emotions, according to which inner, emotional states are the causes of outward behavior. When doing therapy, it is common to hear clients talk about "emotions" and use the verb "to feel" in a variety of puzzling ways that primarily suggest that "emotions" are the cause of undesirable behaviors. Therapists, in workshops, seminars, and professional articles, generally agree with this perspective and frequently talk about "emotions . . . that initiate action," that "provide impulses to act in certain ways" (Kiser, Piercy, & Lipchik, 1993,

p. 235). This leads to treating "emotions" like things—like engines (i.e., reification)—or to use predicates normally applicable only to human beings (i.e., the homunculus fallacy). Emotions become little green men inside us that get us to do things we do not necessarily want to do. Thus, the context in which the "emotions" are felt becomes lost, that is, an inner process, one that is seen as a trigger for behaviors, is detached from those very behaviors.

> It often happens that we only become aware of the important facts if we suppress the question "why?"; and then in the course of our investigations these facts lead us to an answer (PI, #471).

The question "why?" is a favorite among therapists, clients, professors, students, and many other puzzled people. The question "Why?" is rather ambiguous; it is not clear whether an answer giving a reason or a cause will satisfy the asker. Certainly within the behavioral sciences and among therapists, at least since Freud's day, a causal statement is the desired (and scientific) answer.

> Then psychology treats of behaviour, not of the mind?
>
> What do psychologists record?—What do they observe? Isn't it the behaviour of human beings, in particular their utterances? But these are not about behavior (PI, p. 179).

Chapter 10

Questions, Misconceptions, and Joys

Why does SFBT ignore people's problems? How can you help anyone if you don't talk about what's wrong?

Sometimes SFBT is portrayed as an approach that does not permit the discussion of problems. Nothing could be further from the truth. In fact, the transcripts included in this book should provide ample evidence to counter this misconception. Carl tells Insoo about the troubles in his family and his desperation the night before the interview. Margaret describes her drug addiction, violent relationship, and "lying" to the family she is living with in her session with Yvonne. And as Robert and his mother talk with Steve, they describe Robert's stomach pain, seeming lack of motivation, and difficulty attending school. No attempt is made in any of these interviews to prevent a client from talking about his or her concerns. In fact, creating a space for or "honoring" the problem is vital to therapy if clients are to feel that the therapist understands their predicament and is interested in helping. When clients describe a problematic feeling or situation, the therapist asks some version of the question, "How do you want that feeling/thought/behavior to be different?" Talking about what people want will almost always be talking about the problem because clients will be describing the difference between the problem and what they want. Thus, when we talk about what clients want, on a phenomenological level, the clients are still talking about their problems, and the pain and suffering associated with them can be validated while still exploring goals and exceptions. Where SFBT differs from other approaches is that solution-focused therapists devote most of their energy to eliciting a rich description of the client's *solution* rather than to producing increasingly detailed descriptions of the problem.

There are a number of reasons for this stance. First, as the client develops a more complex and detailed description of his or her solution, avenues for reaching that solution state are likely to emerge. Margaret, for instance, notes that evidence of a solution in her life would be waking up and not immediately thinking about her former boyfriend. In place of such thoughts would be thoughts of getting a job. Thus, Margaret both articulates her solution and begins to see avenues for reaching it. When the client develops her own path, the motivation to walk it is built in and the therapist doesn't need to "cheerlead" her into following a plan that the therapist feels is best.

A second reason to focus on solution descriptions is that problem descriptions often become routinized and monolithic language structures that obscure the perception of novel or contradictory data. For instance, the label "depression" can become an all-encompassing description leading one to attend primarily to evidence that one is depressed. Periods of tiredness, moments of discouragement, relationship faux pas, nettling irritation at small slights, etc., are granted foreground status while hopeful thoughts about the future, small accomplishments, satisfying interactions, and moments of contentment are either ignored completely or dismissed as naive or untrustworthy because they do not corroborate the description of depression. Helping the client develop a solution description provides a linguistic structure in which such experiences no longer must be dismissed. Rather, they now seem to be important and trustworthy and can be embraced as evidence of the solution coming to pass. To continue the example of Margaret, the next time she awakens and realizes after a time that she did not immediately think of her boyfriend, she can now embrace this as evidence that she is moving toward a solution and not as a few moments of denial in her continuing addiction to her boyfriend.

How can you have a therapy that doesn't deal with feelings?

Chapter 9 is devoted to the issue of emotion and SFBT and the reader is referred to that chapter for a fuller discussion. In short, however, SFBT has gained a reputation for being an approach that doesn't deal with emotions. Like the alleged prohibition against discussing problems, denying or discouraging emotion in clients is a misconception. At the same time, however, SFBT doesn't promote the discussion of feeling either. Emotion arises as the client needs or wants it to arise and the SFBT therapist acknowledges it but typically does not try to elicit a more detailed description of what the feeling is nor what the client attributes it to ("Why do you think you feel that way?"). No SFBT therapist would discourage a client from expressing feelings. To do so, if nothing else, would be disrespectful. At the same time, SFBT therapists will not ask clients to add more and more language to a description of an inner emotional state and to speculate about its presumed cause and effects ("What do you think makes you so sad? When you feel sad, what other feelings do you have?"). Instead, SFBT suggests that situating emotional states in outward actions and contexts is more useful as this is where clients want change to be manifest. In addition, talking about emotions as if they existed independent of actions, behaviors, and relationships with other people mystifies emotion—setting an arbitrary boundary between inner and outer worlds that violates the wholeness of our experience.

Questions that might be asked to make this shift in focus include: "What would you see yourself doing that would tell you that you are happier?"—a behavioral indicator of a change in the inner state. A contextual question might be something like: "How would your wife know you were feeling better? What would she see?" SFBT sees emotional states as intimately connected with actions that take place in an external context. While SFBT therapists may not discuss emotions in the way they are traditionally discussed in therapy, their careful attention to the external indicators of emotional change gives clients a chance to develop a more detailed sense of the markers of emotional change that direct them to observe the outside world rather than continue to focus inward. Chapter 9 explores these issues in greater depth.

PARAMETERS OF THE NONEXPERT STANCE

You assume that people always know what to do. Many of my clients don't have a clue. Sometimes you have to tell people what they need to do. Isn't that what people pay therapists for?

In debating the issue of what differentiates SFBT from other approaches, one seasoned solution-focused therapist suggested that one would not see a solution-focused therapist giving advice. This brought a quizzical look to Insoo's face. "What?" she said. "You mean that if you knew something that would help the client, you wouldn't tell them?" The solution-focused conviction that clients have the information they need to design and achieve a desired outcome can sometimes be taken to mean that the therapist never offers ideas, suggestions, or alternatives during a therapeutic conversation. This isn't necessarily the case. However, there are two caveats about advice-giving from a SFBT perspective.

First, compared to skill-training or deficit-remediating approaches, advice-giving doesn't happen often in SFBT. The client is the first and foremost authority on where they want to go and how to get there. In teaching communication skills, for instance, the skill-training therapist takes almost total charge of providing the direction the client is to follow. A solution-focused therapist would spend much more time eliciting examples of the client's experiences of communicating well and helping the client see what he or she did in those instances.

Second, the SFBT therapist's suggestions are simply that—suggestions. They are offered tentatively, as alternatives the client may adopt or discard depending on whether or not they fit. The therapist may even distance himself or herself from the suggestion by attributing it to others ("Some other clients have found it useful to seek out a lawyer under these circumstances. Does that make sense for you?") The client remains in charge of the goals of therapy. This differs greatly from more prescriptive approaches that depend on the client adopting the ideas the therapist provides.

Therapists, by and large, are very generous people with a genuine desire to help others. Oftentimes we express this desire by generously sharing our many ideas about things we think can make a difference in our clients' lives. Sadly, most of our good ideas are not new to our clients. They have heard them before. If we persist in our generosity, the situation can easily become a polite (sometimes not so polite) therapeutic argument where the client rebuts each of our well-intended suggestions with evidence that it is impossible, impractical, or otherwise unacceptable. Further efforts to convince the client only raise the intensity of the argument. Thus, we are better served as therapists by changing our views of what our job is in therapy. Our job is not to think up the right solutions for our clients and convince them to accept them. Our job is to create the conditions under which clients find their own solutions, to help clients look into their hearts to find what they truly want and how they might get there.

Sometimes clients are in denial and need to be confronted about their problems. Doesn't SFBT ignore serious problems when you don't confront people?

Confronting clients is based on the assumption that we are aware of things in our clients' lives that they are not aware of. Thus, we are urged to confront people about the ill effects of their drinking, their anger, their abusive style of parenting, and so forth when we see them. However, confrontation most often moves the client into a defensive stance and the therapist into a frustrated one. It can even backfire. At least one study (Miller, Benefield, & Tonigan, 1993) found that confronting people with alcohol problems about their drinking resulted in more, not less, alcohol use after treatment ended.

What to do, then, when clients appear to be unaware of, or in denial about, harmful situations in their lives? One useful strategy is to ask contextual questions. For instance, "I know you don't see a problem with your temper. However, what do you think your children would like to see different when it comes to expressing angry feelings? How about your wife? Your coworkers?" Asking clients to reflect on others' views of their situation allows them to acknowledge difficulties without immediately "owning" them. Clients are also more likely to effectively and meaningfully "confront" themselves under these circumstances than we might be able to.

What about issues of danger and safety? Do SFBT therapists just ignore issues of safety if the client doesn't bring them up or think they are important?

Again, this is a gross misunderstanding, arising from the assumption that if we do not "address" it, somehow we are ignoring it. Quite the contrary. SFBT has been successfully applied in working with domestic violence offenders (Lee, Sebold, & Uken, 2003), child abuse and neglect investigation work of the child welfare services (Berg & Kelly, 2000), work to train prisoners inside while they are serving time (Walker, Sakai, & Brady, 2006), treatment of substance abusers (Berg & Miller, 1992; Berg & Reuss, 1997; McCollum & Trepper, 2001), and working with those who are found guilty of DUI and many other populations. SFBT is used as a basic policy in operating alternative high schools with remarkable rates of success (Streeter & Franklin, 2002), and even in classrooms of dropout prevention programs in junior and high school special education populations. Suicide prevention programs for suicidal adolescents based on SFBT principles are proven to be effective.

The difference between SFBT and other approaches is that the SFBT therapist does his or her best to use the client's ideas and vision to maintain safety, regardless of the nature of the problems presented by the client and regardless of whether the client has been forced to seek therapy as an alternative to incarceration or worse punishments. Drawing upon the work of Insoo Kim Berg and her colleagues in the field of child abuse and neglect (Berg & Kelly, 2000; De Jong & Berg, 1998), numerous social workers have been trained to ask a series of questions designed to elicit what the client and/or others, including children in danger, would say they want and need to do in order to maintain and increase the level of safety in the situations it is needed most in the client's daily life. Because SFBT is based on the assumption that clients are the experts on their own lives, we always work with their perceived level of safety, no matter how small, and then figure out ways to increase the existing level of safety. Therefore, it becomes the client's solution, not one imposed on the client by outside forces. We believe that telling clients what to do is disrespectful and demeaning to their dignity. In addition, on a pragmatic side, when it is their own idea to change, most people change as much as they can for as long as they can, while when they are forced to change against their will, most people will change as little as possible and for as short a time as possible.

For example, a practitioner working with a woman who wants to return to an abusive relationship may be tempted to see her as unable to make good decisions for herself and/or her children, and may thus succumb to the temptation to lecture, educate, and advocate for her to leave the relationship. Instead, approaching the same situation with a mind-set of wanting to learn about the client's thinking behind such a decision, the therapist might say, "You must have a very good reason for wanting to return to what you described as a very dangerous situation. I wonder what might be your good reason for this?" This approach would open up an entirely different way of learning about her "logical" thinking and about what she sees as important to her and to her children and what she is hoping for herself and her children's future. This approach of opening up options and choices would be much more empowering for the woman in this situation than telling her what she should do. For someone who lives in an abusive situation, the last thing she would want is to have someone else try to impose his or her ideas and solutions on her. In addition, it would amount to adding insult to injury to what are already very demeaning circumstances. We do not believe it is an either/or choice, but both/and, that is, she can maintain her dignity and still make decisions that are good for herself and her children. Therapists need to think in terms of developing a detailed safety plan that fits the client's experience and life realities. In addition, scaling questions can be quite useful to indicate small incremental changes that she can implement, rather than trying to make huge changes at a time when she is most under intense stress.

What about issues of social control such as reporting child abuse?

Having done a great deal of work with the child protective services in several U.S. states and in numerous countries in Europe and Asia, Insoo Kim Berg has adapted and extensively applied the principles of SFBT to working with legally mandated (involuntary) clients.

We need to remember that when we use words such as "social control," there is an implied idea behind the question, that is, the "social control" functions of certain services conflict with SFBT principles of working with the client's agenda. As has been emphasized throughout this book, SFBT advocates for practitioners to work with clients' wishes and desires for better lives, as they imagine them. We have never met clients who indicate to us that they like being "forced to" work with us, nor has Insoo ever heard of a client who loves to be visited by child protective workers as a surprise. When asked what would make their life better a little bit even during the "surprise" visit, most clients usually respond with, "I really have nothing against you personally, you seem like a nice person, but I just want to get you out of my life for good." And of course, it is the service's goal to close the case, when the conditions are appropriate. Therefore, immediately aligning with what clients want and what the agency wants can create a common goal. Certain definite steps must be taken by all sides in order to achieve this common goal of "getting you out of one another's lives." This is where a great deal of negotiation is possible, and much of the good work occurs by listening to the client's idea of how getting you out of his or her life will make the client's life better. It means doggedly following the client's idea of what, when, who, where, and how things will be different, who will notice these changes first, and what their responses would be to these changes.

Even when it is necessary to separate a child from his or her parents who are unable to properly care for the child, there are both respectful ways to do it and demeaning, arrogant, and punitive ways. For example, one can separate a child from the parent "because we both want your child to be safe," or "because you are a bad parent." Most parents or caretakers who are not able to follow the community standard of adequate parenting are painfully aware that they are not measuring up. The important point is to find solutions to these difficulties, not to blame the parents for being inadequate. Insoo never met parents who deliberately want their child's life be worse than what they had. Most parents want their children's lives to be better than what they had, in fact. It is more useful to think of the necessity of their changing as moving up to the common social or community standard, rather than "social control."

SFBT AND OTHER APPROACHES

Isn't SFBT just a version of . . . ?

People who are learning SFBT (or anything new, for that matter), often try to fit it into an existing schema. At workshops, people will ask if SFBT isn't just a version of another therapeutic approach, an approach they typically already know and use. Linking the two fits the new knowledge into an existing framework and gives a sense of comfort and familiarity. While there may be some scholarly reasons to debate the differences and similarities between therapy approaches, fitting SFBT too quickly into an existing schema has some dangers. It will emphasize the similarities while obscuring what may be significant differences. For instance, SFBT is often described as being a version of cognitive-behavioral therapy (CBT). Clearly, SFBT focuses on thoughts and actions as does CBT. However, the prescriptive and directive aspects of CBT stand in stark contrast to SFBT's conviction that clients should choose their own goals and their own paths to achieving them. To think of SFBT as simply a version of CBT may obscure this fundamental difference. The Zen concept of beginner's mind is useful here. It is hard for experts to learn new things because their minds are already full of maps and assumptions about how the world is. Learning something new means displacing some well-loved and familiar concepts. The beginner, on the other hand, brings fewer preconceptions to the task of learning and is likely to see the new information more clearly. We suggest those coming to learn SFBT (or anything else) approach the task with the best version of beginner's mind they can muster. One can always return to the old ways if the new ones prove lacking.

Can I integrate SFBT with . . . ?

This is often a sister question to the previous one. Note that while we have recommended beginner's mind as a good stance for learning a new approach, we have not recommended total amnesia. Many techniques from other approaches can be used to good effect within the SFBT framework. Yvonne, for instance, is trained as an Ericksonian therapist and uses some hypnotic imagery in her delivery of the miracle question in her interview with Margaret. However, any technique that requires a directive or expert stance on the part of the therapist or that compromises the client's ability to choose the direction of therapy is not compatible with SFBT and should not be used if one wishes to maintain a solution-focused stance.

This might be a good time to discuss the process by which people adopt SFBT as their primary therapeutic approach. Pichot and Dolan (2003) propose three levels of adopting SFBT. The first level involves incorporating some solution-focused techniques into an already-existing therapeutic approach. The preexisting approach remains the primary orientation. Thus, a therapist who primarily uses a behavioral approach might treat a client couple's report of a good week as an exception and ask a series of questions about how each member of the couple contributed to this atypical outcome. The therapist might then narrow the focus to inquire how the couple used the conflict resolution skills he or she had been teaching them to achieve a good outcome. Behavioral skill training remains the primary approach, although an exception is noted and expanded.

The second level according to Pichot and Dolan is adopting SBFT techniques and core assumptions as the basis for therapy. In this case, therapy will take on the qualities seen in the transcripts in this book—client-directed and delivered by therapists who eschew the expert role.

Finally, Pichot and Dolan see a level where SFBT core assumptions become a life philosophy—pervading not only one's work in the therapy room but also the way agencies are run, colleagues are dealt with, and lives are lived. Exploring this, of course, is outside the bounds of this book.

MATTERS OF STYLE

All you seem to do is ask questions. Don't clients get irritated with all those questions?

Questions do form a fundamental part of SFBT and it is hard to imagine doing therapy without them. It is important to remember, however, that there are many kinds of questions—differentiated as much by their tone as by their content. Some questions are asked by therapists as a way of teaching clients something the therapist thinks they need to know. For instance, "What do you think will happen to your marriage if you continue to drink a 12-pack every night when you come home from work?" Such a question is not an information-seeking question. Rather, the therapist has a clear idea of what will happen if the client continues to drink and is using a question to try to get the client to say it. Such questions usually leave clients hesitant to answer for fear their answer will be used against them. For instance, answering the question about drinking by saying "My wife will probably leave me" leaves the client open to being told he is pretty foolish to keep drinking. While this may be true, it is hard for the client to acknowledge such a truth to someone who is using the question to prove that he or she knows more about what to do than he does.

On an even more subtle level, whenever we develop our own view of what is best for the client, it will show in our questions. The client is then put into the position of having to reflect on our ideas, or on what we want. It is enough for clients to think about what *they* want without us making their job even tougher. When we succeed in not having an agenda for the client (something we can aspire to but probably never truly achieve), we communicate our confidence in our clients' ability to guide their own lives.

Other questions—and most SFBT questions would likely fall into this category—are sincerely intended to elicit the client's view of things. No assumption is made ahead of time about what a "right" or "better" answer to such a question might be. In his interview with Robert and his mother, Steve asks, "Another related kind of question, okay? How long would it [the stomach pain] have to stay at 7½ to convince you that the improvement was permanent? Or what other ways might—what other things might convince you that it's permanently better?" This seems to be an information-seeking question, a question to which Steve is truly interested in hearing the client's unique response. An answer of "30 minutes" would be just as useful and "true" as an answer of "6 months." Questions that truly seek to help us understand the client's view, without subtly imposing our own, rarely draw angry responses from clients. They may find such questions difficult because they ask about things the client may not have thought about before, but they are unlikely to result in the client being angry at the therapist.

SFBT seems to be a slow-moving approach. Clients have to think about the questions. My agency makes me get a lot of assessment data in a short amount of time. I don't have time to be solution-focused.

Sometimes people think that SFBT has a leisurely or slow pace, and this can be true when clients need to take their time answering some of the questions that are asked. In fact, it is usually a good sign when clients can't immediately answer a question since this means that they have to think in new or unaccustomed ways. At times, this pace can seem to be at odds with the demands of an agency, or with the therapist's own wish to gather a lot of information quickly. We encourage therapists to err on the side of helping clients think! While gathering information is important, giving clients new opportunities to envision their future and begin to make plans to move toward that future is equally, if not more, important. Sometimes therapists, when faced with a long list of client problems, feel that they must cover a lot of material in a session to make sure they have attended to all of the client's concerns. One of the assumptions of brief therapists in general is that small changes made in therapy can generate large ripples of change in the rest of the client's life. Therefore, working hard and carefully to help the client envision and make a small change will likely return more benefit over time than trying to cover a lot of territory quickly but not as well. And, in the process of asking solution-focused questions, much of the needed information will emerge. If an agency protocol demands that certain information be gathered in order for the client to be seen, it may be best to simply tell the client you are setting aside a few minutes at the beginning of the first session to ask required questions, and then you will discuss their concerns in a more conversational way.

I think SFBT is just a Band-Aid. What about deep-seated feelings and problems?

It depends on what you mean by deep. As we noted earlier, SFBT steers away from elaborate descriptions of inner negative states. In the traditional sense, then, SFBT isn't "deep." What SFBT does look at in depth, however, is a deep understanding of the client's everyday life and the changes he or she would like to see there. Paradoxically, this challenges the therapist to stay on the surface in order to develop a deep understanding of the client's life and desired outcome. Doing so is difficult because we have a culturally and professionally entrenched vision that actions in the world spring from separate inner, private states of the individual. Not only does SFBT dispute this assumed connection, it also disputes the distinction between inner and outer and between emotion, cognition, and action. From an SFBT perspective, therefore, coming to a detailed and careful understanding of a client's everyday life is deep.

WHAT IS THE EVIDENCE THAT SFBT WORKS?

Research on SFBT is growing. Gingerich and Eisengart (2000) identified 15 studies that tested the outcome of SFBT. These studies varied in their level of experimental control. Of 5 studies judged to be reasonably well-controlled, all showed significant positive outcomes for SFBT. Gingerich continues to update his review of the outcome studies on his Web site (www.gingerich.net). By 2001, he had identified 18 outcome studies of SFBT, including 7 well-controlled studies. Of the 18 studies, 17 showed positive results for SFBT. While the question about SFBT's effectiveness is still open to some extent, there is certainly growing evidence that it works.

WHAT ARE THE JOYS OF SFBT? COULDN'T A COMPUTER DO IT?

SFBT sounds kind of boring. What's the fun in asking the miracle question over and over again?

Maybe it's a matter of taste. Some people like the flare of a big jazz band while others find a jazz trio more to their liking. While no one can deny that the complex harmonies of a multi-section band are interesting, the endless variation of sounds that emerge from piano, bass, and drums can be equally compelling. Those who are drawn to SFBT may be more like those who enjoy jazz trios. The creativity and art in SFBT comes from learning to work within the frame the approach demands and to help clients create masterpieces from the everyday melodies of their lives. While this approach to therapy may not have the outward intensity of "dance-band" therapy, it is no less creative or satisfying.

What do therapists experience when they do SFBT?

Two of us (EM and TT) have spent several years now training substance abuse counselors to work with families using SFBT. Many of them have expanded their use of the model to include their individual and group work as well. Each time we trained and supervised these folks we noticed a similar phenomenon. After a few months, as they became more comfortable with the model, they began to report a renewed interest in their work and a decreased sense of burnout. One counselor said that attendance at his group sessions for teens had increased dramatically when he turned to helping them think about future successes, not past failures. He was delighted and enjoyed the kids more. Another counselor reported that families seemed reassured and willing to work harder when he acknowledged their areas of strength.

But one January day, a counselor I was supervising summed up this difference very nicely. "This was the best Christmas season I've had in years," she told me. "Before, I was always so worried that one of my clients would relapse. I'd find myself thinking about my clients constantly as I noticed all the temptations around the holidays—office parties, ads everywhere for alcohol, New Year's Eve. This year, I realized that my clients have the skills to avoid relapse and that's a job they have to do. I just kind of relaxed about it. They know what to do."

This was not a counselor who had retreated into the cynical disinterest of burnout. She still cared passionately about her clients. What was different was her increased confidence in them and in the work they had been doing together. SFBT suggests a much more equal partnership between client and therapist, one in which the client does as much or more "heavy lifting" as the therapist. With this shift also can come a more relaxed connection to clients. It's easier to be an interested and compassionate companion for someone on the road to change when you don't feel burdened with the responsibility of their change.

Conclusion

To begin with, we want to thank you for having joined our seminar. We sincerely hope that you have found it useful and will continue to find it useful. We all enjoyed putting it together via watching tapes, having conversations, cooking, eating, drinking wine and beer, writing separately and sometimes together, and a huge bundle of e-mails.

Ever since I met Matthias Varga von Kibed (Professor of logic and philosophy, University of Munich) in 1989, we have had many wide-ranging conversations around Wittgensteinian topics that have convinced me (SdS) more and more that Wittgenstein's way of describing the world—language at work—is very appropriate, highly useful, and quite fitting for solution-focused brief therapists. Some of the results of this continuing conversation are reflected in my view of the usefulness of Wittgenstein's work in describing what we do. As teachers and trainers, the clearer the description we have, the easier it is to help people learn how to do SFBT, thus the interspersal of quotes from Wittgenstein's works in the interview chapters and the chapters on emotions. We thought you might find our adding Wittgenstein's voice to the conversation both interesting and clarifying.

We hope you found the whole seminar useful and that you had some fun, but not too much.

Steve de Shazer
June 2005

References

Berg, I.K. & Dolan, Y. (2001). *Tales of solutions: A collection of hope-inspiring stories*. New York: Norton.
Berg, I.K. & Kelly, S. (2000). *Building solutions in child protective services*. New York: Norton.
Berg, I.K. & Miller, S. (1992). *Working with the problem drinker: A solution-focused approach*. New York: Norton.
Berg, I.K. & Reuss, N. (1997). *Solutions step by step: A substance abuse treatment manual*. New York: Norton.
Bouveresse, J. (1995). *Wittgenstein reads Freud: The myth of the unconscious* (trans. T. Cosman). Princeton: Princeton University Press.
Cade, Brian (1997). E-mail to The Solution-Focused Therapy Mailing List and Network, May 17.
Cantwell, P. & Holmes, S. (1994). Social construction: A paradigm shift for systemic therapy and training. *Australia and New Zealand Journal for Family Therapy, 15(1)*, 17-26.
Caufman, L. (2001). Challenging the family business: The relational dimension. *Scandinavia Journal of Organizational Psychology, 2*, 1-12.
De Jong, P. & Berg, I.K. (1998). *Interviewing for solutions*. Pacific Grove, CA: Brooks/Cole.
de Shazer, S. (1985). *Keys to solution in brief therapy*. New York: Norton.
de Shazer, S. (1988). *Clues: Investigating solutions in brief therapy*. New York: Norton.
de Shazer, S. (1991). *Putting difference to work*. New York: Norton.
de Shazer, S. (1994). *Words were originally magic*. New York: Norton.
de Shazer, S. & Isebaert, L. (2003). The Bruges model: A solution-focused approach to problem drinking. *Journal of Family Psychotherapy, 14*, 43-52.
Dolan, Y. (1991). *Resolving sexual abuse: Solution-focused therapy and Ericksonian hypnosis for adult survivors*. New York: Norton.
Dolan, Y. (1998). *One small step: Moving beyond trauma and therapy to a life of joy*. New York: Papier Mache Press.
Eakes, G., Walsh, S., Markowski, M., Cain, H., & Swanson, M. (1997). Family-centered brief solution-focused therapy with chronic schizophrenia: A pilot study. *Journal of Family Therapy, 19*, 145-158.
Fogelin, R.J. (1996). Wittgenstein's critique of philosophy. In H. Sluga and D.G. Stern (Eds.), *The Cambridge companion to Wittgenstein*. Cambridge: Cambridge University Press.

Gingerich, W.J. & Eisengart, S. (2000). Solution-focused brief therapy: A review of the outcome research. *Family Process, 39*, 477-498.
Glock, H-J. (1996). *A Wittgenstein dictionary*. Oxford: Blackwell.
Godzich, W. (1986). Introduction in de Man, P. *The resistance to theory*. Minneapolis: University of Minnesota Press.
Haley, J. (1973). *Uncommon therapy: The psychiatric techniques of Milton H. Erickson, MD.* New York: Norton.
Kiser, D.J., Piercy, F.P., & Lipchik, E. (1993). The integration of emotion in solution-focused therapy. *Journal of Marital and Family Therapy, 19,* 233-242.
Lee, M.Yi, Sebold, J., & Uken, A. (2003). *Solution-focused treatment of domestic violence offenders: Accountability for solutions.* London & New York: Oxford University Press.
McCollum, E.E. & Trepper, T.S. (2001). *Creating family solutions for substance abuse.* New York: The Haworth Press.
Miller, W.R., Benefield, R.G., & Tonigan, J.S. (1993). Enhancing motivation for change in problem drinking: A controlled comparison of two therapist styles. *Journal of Consulting and Clinical Psychology, 61*, 455-461.
Pichot, T. & Dolan, Y. (2003). *Solution-focused brief therapy: Its effective use in agency settings*. New York: The Haworth Press.
Rhodes, J. & Ajmal, Y. (2001). *Solution-focused thinking in schools*. London: BT Press.
Staten, H. (1984). *Wittgenstein and Derrida*. Lincoln: University of Nebraska Press.
Streeter, C.L. & Franklin, C. (2002). Standards for school social work in the 21st century. In A.R. Roberts and G.J. Greene (Eds.), *Social workers' desk reference*. New York: Oxford University Press.
Stroll, A. (2002). *Wittgenstein*. Oxford: Oneworld Publications.
Sulloway, F.J. (1979). *Freud, biologist of the mind: Beyond the psychoanalytic legend.* New York: Basic Books.
Walker, L., Sakai, T., & Brady, K. (2006). Restorative circles: A reentry planning process for Hawaii inmates, *Federal Probation Journal 70(2),* 1-9.
Watzlawick, P., Weakland, J., & Fish, R. (1974). *Change: Principles of problem formation and problem resolution*. New York: Norton.
Weiner-Davis, M. (1993). *Divorce-busting: A step-by-step approach to making your marriage loving again*. New York: Fireside.
Williams, M. (2002). *Wittgenstein, mind and meaning: Toward a social conception of mind.* London: Routledge.

Key to the works of Ludwig Wittgenstein

BBB Wittgenstein, L. (1958). *The blue and brown books*. Cambridge: Basil Blackwell.
CV Wittgenstein, L. (1984). *Culture and value* (trans. P Winch). Chicago: University of Chicago Press.
L & C Wittgenstein, L. (1972). *Lectures & conversations on aesthetics, psychology, and religious belief.* Ed. C. Barrett. Berkeley: University of California Press.

LWPP Wittgenstein, L. (1982). *Last writings on the philosophy of psychology*. Volume One (trans. C.G. Luckhardt & M.A.E. Aue). Eds. G.H. von Wright & Heikki Nyman. Chicago: University of Chicago Press.

PI Wittgenstein, L. (1958). *Philosophical investigations* (trans. G.E.M. Anscombe). New York: Macmillan.

PR Wittgenstein, L. (1975). *Philosophical remarks* (trans. R. Hargreaves & R. White). Ed. R. Rhess. Chicago: University of Chicago Press.

RPP1 Wittgenstein, L. (1980). *Remarks on the philosophy of psychology, Vol. 1* (trans. G.E.M. Anscombe). Eds. G.E.M. Anscombe & G.H. von Wright. Chicago: University of Chicago Press.

RPP2 Wittgenstein, L. (1980). *Remarks on the philosophy of psychology, Vol. II* (trans. G.E.M. Anscombe). Eds. G.E.M. Anscombe & G.H. von Wright. Chicago: University of Chicago Press.

T Wittgenstein, L. (1962). *Tractatus logico-philosophicus* (trans. C.K. Ogden). London: Routledge.

Z Wittgenstein, L. (1970). *Wittgenstein: Zettel* (trans G.E.M. Anscombe & G.H. von Wright). Ed. G.E.M. Anscombe. Berkeley: University of California Press.

Index

For Product Safety Concerns and Information please contact our EU
representative GPSR@taylorandfrancis.com
Taylor & Francis Verlag GmbH, Kaufingerstraße 24, 80331 München, Germany

www.ingramcontent.com/pod-product-compliance
Ingram Content Group UK Ltd.
Pitfield, Milton Keynes, MK11 3LW, UK
UKHW022313250926
475702UK00046B/755
9780367622435